Traditional Family Values
and Substance Abuse

THE PLENUM SERIES IN CULTURE AND HEALTH

SERIES EDITORS:

Richard M. Eisler and Sigrid Gustafson
Virginia Polytechnic Institute and State University, Blacksburg, Virginia

HANDBOOK OF DIVERSITY ISSUES IN HEALTH PSYCHOLOGY
  Edited by Pamela M. Kato and Traci Mann

TRADITIONAL FAMILY VALUES AND SUBSTANCE ABUSE
  Mary Cuadrado and Louis Lieberman

Traditional Family Values and Substance Abuse

The Hispanic Contribution to an Alternative Prevention and Treatment Approach

MARY CUADRADO

University of South Florida at Sarasota
Sarasota, Florida

and

LOUIS LIEBERMAN

John Jay College of Criminal Justice
New York, New York

Kluwer Academic / Plenum Publishers
New York   Boston   Dordrecht   London   Moscow

Library of Congress Cataloging-in-Publication Data

Traditional family values and substance abuse/edited by Mary Cuadrado and Louis Lieberman.
   p.   cm. — (The Plenum series in culture and health)
   Includes bibliographical references (p.   ) and index.
   ISBN 0-306-46619-8
   1. Puerto Ricans—Drug use—United States.   2. Puerto Ricans—Alcohol use—United
States.   3. Puerto Ricans—United States x Family relationships.   4. Puerto Ricans—United
States x Attitudes.   5. Alcoholism—United States—Public opinion.   6. Public
opinion—United States.   I. Cuadrado, Mary.   II. Lieberman, Louis.   III. Series.

HV524.E85 T73 2001
362.29'12'089687295—dc21

                                                                                   2001038595

ISBN 0-306-46619-8

©2002 Kluwer Academic / Plenum Publishers
233 Spring Street, New York, New York 10013

http://www.wkap.nl/

10 9 8 7 6 5 4 3 2 1

A C.I.P. record for this book is available from the Library of Congress

Printed in the United States of America

To my parents,
Juan Cuadrado Falcón and María Caridad Almánzar-Cuadrado,
who, through love and example, taught me the value of tradition
(Para mis padres, los cuales por medio de su amor y ejemplo
me enseñaron el valor de la tradición).

—M.C.

To my son Joel and daughter-in-law Celia,
the proud and happy parents of my brilliant, beautiful,
and talented twin baby grandchildren, Ben and Sarah,
who will grow up to experience the joys and wisdom of tradition.

—L.L.

ACKNOWLEDGMENTS

We are greatly indebted to Dr. Gerald Gurin, Principal Investigator on the Survey of Drinking Behavior, Norms, and Problems of Puerto Rican Adults project, and to the Fordham University Hispanic Research Center for providing the raw data used in this volume. Without their generosity, this study would not have been possible.

We are grateful to Eliot Werner, Editor, and Richard M. Eisler, Series Editor, at Kluwer Academic/Plenum Publishing for their continuing support, suggestions, and encouragement.

We also are happy to acknowledge the influence of our good friend Dr. Ruth Westheimer who over these many years has personified the importance of ethnic and religious traditions as a source of strength and growth. It was at the New School for Social Research where Dr. Westheimer and one of the authors first met as students in the late 1950s. We were both greatly influenced by the graduate "Faculty in Exile" where many of the theoretical problems involving conflicts, adaptations, and integration of immigrants were explored, based on firsthand experiences, by Professor Alfred Schutz and his colleagues. Their influence and theoretical insights will be seen throughout this volume.

TABLE OF CONTENTS

INTRODUCTION

The main goal of this volume is to show that adherence to a more traditionalist view of one's culture has the socially desired consequence of inhibiting the emergence of deviant behaviors such as alcohol and other forms of substance abuse. By introducing and defining the concept of "traditionalism" we do not mean the narrow conception of obedience to laws that may prohibit illicit drug use or the adherence to traditional norms that regulate the circumstances of alcohol and other substance use, as important as both of these may be, but rather an outlook on everyday life that is comprehensive and not restricted to specific norms. Among the unique contributions of this volume is the demonstration that, *even in the absence of clear regulatory laws and norms, persons who are more traditional in their outlook and social relations are less likely to engage in deviant behavior.*

The findings presented in this volume derive from a carefully designed stratified area probability sample of 1084 interviews with Puerto Ricans in the New York City area. Instruments that tap the broader concept of traditionalism through an analysis of traditional gender norms are developed and validated based on the data collected in this study. In addition instruments to measure acculturation, alcohol and substance use, alcohol-related problems, fatalism, and others were developed for this volume and used to help understand the relationships between traditionalism and the inhibition of substance abuse.

The traditional values discussed in this volume are essentially family values; that is, the values that help define the role of husband and wife toward each other and the raising of children on a day-to-day basis. These are gender-based values reflecting traditional Hispanic role assignments and have no direct relationship to alcohol or illicit drug use but only to how much a person believes in and acts out traditional values and behaviors. Yet, when we examine the degree of commitment to traditional family values, we find that low commitment is indicative of the likelihood of acting in a socially undesirable manner in the area of substance use.

Among the conclusions reached in this volume is that, political rhetoric notwithstanding, it is *not the promotion of specific values* that must be promulgated in order to prevent certain individual and social ills but *rather it is the promotion of a "sense of tradition" itself* that is needed. Our use of the phrase "sense of tradition" is derived from the pride and knowledge about the norms and culture of one's familial ethnic group, for it is *ethnic pride and identification* that may provide, as suggested by the psychologist Kurt Lewin (1948), "a firm ground on which to stand," i.e., a strong bond linking one's self to a larger community. Individual behavior and interpersonal choices are then more likely to be made with respect to and agreement with this community reference group.

We believe that the findings presented in this volume suggest a new variety of ethnotherapy that can be used as an ancillary treatment and prevention modality for substance abuse as well as many other aspects of socially undesirable behaviors in the Hispanic populations. In addition, the development of measures of traditionalism are explicitly presented, enabling others to modify them for ethnic groups other than Hispanic, so that a culturally appropriate use of ethnotherapy may be employed specific to each ethnic group.

This focus on a return to tradition and traditional values projected in this volume does not place emphasis on the repressive, nonfunctional, and discarded elements of any particular tradition but rather draws from the ego-enhancing elements. For example, among Puerto Rican males, in keeping with Hispanic tradition, the emphasis would be away from the destructive aspects of *machismo* and toward the positive images of the traditional *caballero*—the supportive gentleman. Similarly, among females, the destructive syndrome of *marianismo* (submissiveness toward males, passive acceptance of destiny) may be replaced by *hembrismo*—the assertive and independent woman or *la nueva marianista*. The latter is a role proposed by Gil and Vazquez (1996) based on the constructive and supportive elements of the Puerto Rican wife and mother that draws from traditional concepts and values even for the acculturated woman. At bottom, this is a study of specific family values reflecting a larger value orientation—traditionalism—and how traditionalism may affect substance abuse. What, however, do we mean by family values?

A dominant and recurring theme of the political campaigns for the last decade and more has been the importance of returning to and emphasizing "family values." This theme is reiterated not only by Democratic and Republican Party spokespersons but also by members of the clergy, social reformers, and a myriad of other social commentators. For many years now, members of these and other segments of society have referred to "the loss of traditional family values" to account for a variety of vaguely formulated theories as to the causes of crime, illicit sexuality, underemployment, divorce, out-of-wedlock pregnancies, and, substance abuse, among other social ills. Attempts at precision in meaning of this term are virtually nonexistent in the media or in social science literature. Examples of how a "loss" of "family values" produces socially undesirable behavior in any semblance of a causal relationship has been neither explained nor demonstrated with research data. On the other hand, there are some accepted examples of how values may prevent widespread problems in communities, e.g., cultures and subcultures that encourage drinking but forbid drunkenness or religions that prohibit the use of beverage alcohol (Pittman, 1967). However, it would be foolish to proceed in a deterministic fashion by assuming that a missing value is necessarily the culprit for a corresponding social ill, or its opposite, the projection of a "bad" value, that causes one to go astray. The notion that "evil begets evil" and that for every socially undesirable consequence there is a pathological or dysfunctional family or singular cause is naive and often diversionary. This "evil begets evil" notion often stems from faulty reasoning due to the *post hoc ergo propter hoc* fallacy, i.e., if a consequence appears after an apparently related event, it must be due to that event. If there are any lessons to be derived from an examination of the socially harmful consequences of a breakdown in family or traditional values, it first must be demonstrated that it is the absence of those specific values that results in the behaviors we wish to avoid rather than a myriad of other possible influences or determinants.

At the heart of the problem of establishing reliable data to examine cause and effect or other statistical relationships is the issue of definition: how do we operationalize the concept of family values? Are the societal discussants referring to *functional* social values manifested within and by families, e.g., role definitions and socially acceptable attitudes or behaviors by family members, or rather do they mean the *structural* social values of having a traditional nuclear family, monogamous and intact, heterosexual, and babies born only in wedlock as Dan Quayle (Quayle & Medved, 1996) has stated? Both may be inferred from the sentiments and contexts. The concept of "family values" has been even further complicated by suggestions that it also means refraining from excessive exposure of the public to visual and audio media deemed violent, vulgar, sexist or salacious, as suggested by Senator Joseph Lieberman and former Drug Czar William Bennett.

Quite often, the phrase "family values" appears to be interchangeable or even synonymous with "traditional values." However, the concept of traditional values might be less politically useful because it begs the question, "whose tradition?" Nonetheless, traditional values might have a greater potential for analysis and research testing than family values. This is because the phrase "traditional values" is often understood and embraced, whether followed or not, by most members of a society and is embodied in the literature, folkways, norms, and laws of a people, e.g., the major elements of the Protestant work ethic, the eastern European Jewish tradition, the Navajo "way," or the Hispanic tradition. We frequently use and seem to understand correctly the concept of tradition and sometimes even accept the validity of differences in traditions. Most people seem to understand that institutions have their own traditions, e.g., historical traditions within a particular college, religious group, or military service. Many members of our society are aware that people in different segments of society live out the controlling and motivating force of their traditions as in the representation of *shtetl* tradition portrayed in *Fiddler on the Roof* or in the Amish community. On the other hand, for most Americans, family values and traditions *within* families may differ from family to family since there is no single cohesive set of family norms in the United States. This often makes it difficult to comprehend, let alone accept what the other person means by family values. It may be easier to see and understand the concept of family values when it is attached to a tradition. We can observe a much more clearly defined and mostly cohesive set of family values in ethnic groups such as the Hassidic or Amish populations than in the core culture or white Anglo-Saxon Protestant (WASP) families who usually do not center their entire lifestyle around a religious theme that demarcates them from other groups. When we examine the clearest illustrations of traditional family values, usually found in the United States among the more fundamentalist religious groups, we find considerable similarities of values with respect to male authority, the role of women, the place of children, the deemphasis on material goods and pursuit of pleasures, as well as the greater emphasis on the importance of religious authority.

These values often present a confusing picture to outsiders, who may have difficulty in reconciling, for example, how the traditional family norms and values of Hassidic Jews in upstate New York often have more in common with fundamentalist Christians than with families in the Reformed or Conservative Jewish communities and yet still can be categorized along with these Reformed and Conservatives as Jews.

To further complicate this discussion, Americans of different political persuasions, from left to right, appear to believe that the less the intrusion of society and social control on the individual family, the better off will be all families and society. Thus, there is congressional (and some public) resistance to a national day care system as well as to national education standards and content for fear of governmental infusion of values. This apparent contradiction—that we should all have the "right" family values to ameliorate social ills but that family values should not be standardized and imposed on families—would appear to negate any impact of the utility of family values as a concept to be taught and supported to prevent or alleviate social ills.

In order to understand the relationship between family values and substance abuse (or violence or unwanted teenage pregnancies or any other socially undesirable consequence) it is necessary to first understand how we use the term "values" in this study. Our definitions and usage of the terms values, morals and ethics will follow the argument developed by Westheimer and Lieberman (1988).

In brief, values represent the worth, the emphasis, the "value" we place on a particular behavior or symbol or material object relative to something else. An implicit assumption in our usage of the term "values" is that they often influence or even determine the choices that individuals make in specific social situations to engage in or refrain from action. However, social values, particularly those we call traditional values, derive from broader considerations of morals and ethics within a social and historical context. Thus, for a better understanding of how we use this concept throughout this volume, we briefly present what we mean by morals, ethics, and values. Where do they come from and what changes are taking place? In a world of ever-increasing and ever-changing choices, what role do they play in shaping our attitudes and guiding our behaviors?

By morals, we mean a set of lofty principles, usually given to us through the ages by our great religious leaders and philosophers and which have withstood the test of time. These are the guidelines that serve as the bases for determining right from wrong in situations that are not always clear to us. Sociologists have called these "moral norms," that is, rules for moral behavior that have been with us for a long time and are approved by the institution out of which they emerged—the institution of religion.

Because of the emphasis our society places on the separation of church and state many religious norms have become embodied in our secular laws, such as in the criminal codes that define crime in each state. Also, some moral norms that at one time reflected only religious views have been modified by state laws because of different religious interpretations as to whether they are right or wrong. Abortion laws and adultery laws are two examples. Other traditional religious moral norms have been questioned in light of contemporary science and knowledge not available to those in biblical times, e.g., the issue of homosexuality.

Ethics are the practical ways of making decisions so that we can determine whether a particular behavior we are uncertain about is right or wrong according to a moral code. Ethical considerations are necessary because the morality of a specific social behavior cannot be judged as an isolated act; we also must consider the social context in which it occurs. Ethics help us evaluate the morality of social behaviors by taking other information into consideration. Take killing, for example. The Bible commands us not to kill. If one person takes the life of another, it may be difficult to judge the morality or immorality of that act unless we know the ethical context within which it is done, for example, protecting ones'

self or family from a predator, law enforcement in the appropriate
conduct of duty, defending ones' nation from invaders, and so forth.

Values are related to but are not the same as morals or ethics. They
are, as discussed above, the "value" or importance we place on specific
day-to-day actions or material things or any creations of a culture. As
simply stated in the foreword to *A Question of Values* (Peck, 1990), they
are "the beliefs that guide our everyday speech and conduct and make
us what we are, (and) how we should respond." It would be simple if
there were a consistency between values and morals, but sometimes
there is a problem relating the two. Interpretations of morality, usually
presented by local authority figures and reinforced by local reference
groups, especially peer groups, are not homogeneous in a pluralistic,
diverse, and geographically complicated society such as the United
States. The love of guns in one community may seem just as moral as the
abhorrence of guns in another. Both groups may adhere to the same
Judeo-Christian moral belief system but are separated by another
element that mediates morals and ethics: tradition. Thus, to the concept
of values, we must append the concept of tradition to help clarify what
one means by values. When individuals believe that they are adhering to
their traditions and the traditions of their family and past generations,
they are more likely to feel moral and believe that they are behaving
ethically since it is reinforced by parents and grandparents. If they have
become "marginal" to their ethnic group, their sense of insecurity can be
very damaging, as Kurt Lewin (1948) has aptly portrayed in his essay
Bringing up the Jewish Child:

> The marginal men and women are in somewhat the same position as an
> adolescent who is no longer a child and certainly does not want to be a
> child any longer, but who knows at the same time that he is not really
> accepted as a grown-up. This uncertainty about the ground on which he
> stands and the group to which he belongs often makes the adolescent loud,
> restless, at once timid and aggressive, over-sensitive and tending to go to
> extremes, over-critical of others and himself. (p. 181)

This firm "ground on which he stands" is a powerful and positive force, but when values are focused less on traditional group identification and more on contemporary peer group influence, then individuals can feel and claim a high moral position even when their actions run counter to the moral beliefs of their parents, religion, and community. This helps to explain the strange phenomenon of persons, particularly young persons, who say that they have their "own moral code," and believe that it is just as moral as the next person's.

Values influence nearly every aspect of our social behavior, from the very mundane to the most far-reaching. The career we choose, the kind of car we drive, the type of people with whom we associate, and even the sorts of food we eat are all reflections of our values. Indeed, when we try to understand social behavior, we find that values are often more influential factors than morals or ethics in shaping our day-to-day behavior. This is true even when we are aware that our values may be in conflict with the moral standards that we are supposed to subscribe to by virtue of our religious upbringing. Often this can be understood by realizing that values may be more tied to feelings, impulses, and irrational forces in the human psyche that are related to the particular situational experience and how we are perceived by other people. The values we project to others—idealistic, materialistic, aesthetic, and other values—are often the bases for how we project *ourselves* to others and want them to think of us. In this way, values are very active in our daily lives, while moral codes may be learned and remain dormant in the absence of continuous social reinforcement by the people around us, our peers, and significant others. Therefore, it appears that values, which are often very changeable, can have more of a day-to-day influence over us than our moral and ethical beliefs.

Most people assume that everyone has been taught and knows a moral code but may choose to abandon it. We frequently hear from politicians and religious leaders that as a civilized nation of laws and rules we must believe in these "traditional values"; that there are basic "moral truths" that we should accept. The problem is that they rarely specify whose "traditional values."

Why should this be so much of a problem? Why can we not do just as our parents did? Because we believe no society in the history of humankind has provided a milieu in which people grow up with as many alternatives for social behavior as we find in the societies of Western culture today and in the United States in particular. Why is this so? Because freedom of choice and variations in social behavior depend on the awareness of available alternatives. In other words, if you believe that you may only choose between job A or job B because you think that you are not eligible for any other positions, you will pick only A or B or nothing at all. But on the other hand if you know that there are people with the same background and brains as you who are also able get jobs C to Z, any one of those job choices can become an option for you. Deciding which job would be best for you requires a different approach to the problem than merely gaining access to information about alternative opportunities. For immigrant groups, coming to mainland United States means for them to be confronted with a set of choices inconceivable back home. Here, there is group support not only for traditional back-home ethics and values but also for the opposite ones. This is particularly true for Hispanic women and men compared with previous immigrant groups who were urged and expected to become "Americanized" and reject the "old country" ways.

A particular concern of society and the focus of this volume comes from the substance abuse area: We may not like the presence of alcohol, heroin, or cocaine in our society today, but we are aware that for now we are free to choose to use these drugs or not. Furthermore, because we are also free to be oblivious to or rationalize the consequences of our choices, we may make the wrong and destructive choice. Are there clear and unequivocal community guidelines to help us, particularly younger persons, to make the correct choices other than the socially contrived legal issues or the extreme and overly dramatic health consequences approach presented in TV ads? Unfortunately, there are not any clear guidelines in the society as a whole with respect to type, frequency, and amount of alcohol and drug use, which has forced some well-intentioned people to engage in campaigns such as "Just Say No to Drugs." We think this approach is insulting to the intelligence of young persons, since it implies a basis for the decision making that denies them the ability to make choices. It says in effect, "Just say no because *we* tell you to." Fortunately and perhaps even in spite of our admonitions most people of all ages are able to resist the temptations of serious substance abuse. Is this because of the existence of specific proscriptive norms as with Hispanic women and alcohol or some other controlling influences in the absence of these proscriptive norms? In this connection, the resistances of many Hispanic men to alcohol abuse, even in traditional communities, appears despite apparent cultural support or at least tolerance that lends itself to excessive and problematic drinking.

It is often difficult to distinguish between substance use, substance misuse, and substance abuse as distinct and different concepts since in this country even the most minimal or isolated use of marijuana or cocaine is labeled as substance abuse. The problem is even more difficult when the substance involved is alcohol since definitions are based not on the use of the substance but on the consequences of the use or the inappropriateness of time or place, criteria not used for other drugs. This conceptual difficulty is especially aggravated when attempting to discuss drinking among Hispanics. For traditional women, being caught having even one drink in proscribed settings such as bars may evoke extreme labeling and condemnation for behavior that most Anglos consider acceptable and nondeviant; nevertheless, the behavior would more correctly be considered as "misuse" than "abuse." Conversely, for men, drinking levels and outcomes may be considered "normal" and typical in traditional Hispanic communities but judged as "alcohol abuse" from an Anglo perspective. Thus, we will attempt to be consistent and use the term "abuse" to represent the more severe behaviors as seen from a

Hispanic perspective, while using "misuse" to represent the more culturally inappropriate behaviors. We acknowledge that this distinction is not perfect nor will it satisfy all critics.

Our approach in this volume is to demonstrate through research data analysis that traditional value conceptions may be much simpler and yet more powerful than has been understood. If we accept the idea that the traditional values of a community include family values, then attempts at analyzing the utility of adhering to specific types of values or norms as a prophylaxis against certain social ills may be more easily researched and discussed, since there already is a body of knowledge concerning the values of different ethnic groups. This presents a clear methodological problem. It is impossible to ignore the fact that we have vastly different communities in the United States based on ethnic, religious, racial, and political identities. If we are to understand which traditional values are important and how they affect social behavior, it seems reasonable that we will have to proceed on a group by group basis. That is, to examine the effect of "traditional family values" we must look separately at each group's values. This volume focuses on one Hispanic group—the mainland Puerto Ricans.

It is a commonly held belief by Hispanics and Anglos alike that traditional Hispanic cultures have had socially explicit and rigid controls over the behavior of women. It has been suggested, for example, that these norms were instrumental in preventing Hispanic women from becoming involved in deviant behavior (Aguirre-Molina, 1991; Trotter, 1985). Similarly, *machismo* stereotypes and norms are often cited to help explain male excess and sexist behaviors. However, as Hispanic women and men move to the United States, it may be possible that the strength of these norms weakens due to the lack of traditional community support for them in an Anglo or mixed society. It is plausible to suggest that a weakening of these traditional role norms may result in an increase in deviant behavior for these women and perhaps a weakening of consequences for men no longer under the scrutiny of small communities. These changes may include departures from culturally acceptable drinking patterns as well as the use of illegal substances and engagement in antisocial behavior. Thus, the consequences of the loss of traditional prescriptive and proscriptive normative controls may be seen as possibly due to the removal or weakening of those factors (norms) that inhibit for women or exacerbate for men the development of substance abuse, criminal, and other deviant behaviors and attitudes.

In this volume, we will examine the proposition that the differences found in substance use and abuse behavior and attitudes among Puerto Ricans living in the United States are based on adherence to a strong identity to Puerto Rican tradition as manifested in the Puerto Rican family. In consideration of the fact that levels of adherence to traditional norms for Hispanics are affected by the process of acculturation when living in mainland United States, we also will examine the question of whether it is the degree of acculturation alone, or whether the degree of acculturation in combination with the loss of traditional ethnic values, or even whether the loss of traditional values alone provides the best explanation for drinking and drug use behaviors and consequences among Puerto Rican women and men.

In sum, the concepts involved in traditional family values and their relationships to morality, ethics, and socially undesirable behaviors need to be discussed within the context of different value structures based on different religions and ethnicities. The relationships between tradition, family, and values have general common threads running through all societies but need to be understood separately for each group. We have chosen to view the Puerto Rican community on the mainland as our social laboratory so as to examine the consequences of a breakdown in certain traditional family values and how this may impact on substance abuse. In the Puerto Rican society, as in other homogeneous populations, traditional community values are best illustrated by family values, most of which are clearly delineated and are expressed through the attitudes and interactions of members of the family.

During the past century, the Hispanic migrations to the United States have been to communities that are less supervised, with the consequent weakening of ties to parental value systems. However, for some migrants, the lure of different and more open values did not become attractive. We will examine why some controls seem more acceptable for some persons than for others. Why do some norms (rules) serve as guidelines and "brakes" so that they help people conform to the traditional expectations of their groups while other norms do not?

This volume begins with a profile of the mainland Puerto Ricans and the problem of acculturation in an Anglo society. In Chapter 3, we discuss the measurement and dimensions of traditionalism. Chapters 4 and 5 present an analysis of alcohol and drug use and abuse patterns and problems in the mainland Puerto Rican community. The relationships between acculturation, traditionalism, background factors, and substance abuse are explored in Chapters 6 and 7. The remainder of the volume addresses possible paths to a more comprehensive social approach based on elements of success found in ethnic approaches to treatment. The value of tradition rather than traditional values is the key element in our approach to ethnicity-based programs and the pride and commitment to one's traditions can be considered as an ancillary treatment modality. We believe that this approach may be seen as a basis to be built on in the various secular and Anglo communities of the wider populations for treatment of a variety of socially undesirable behaviors. They are an affirmation of the principle that conventional and conformist behaviors are more a product of internal mechanisms than external social controls.

CHAPTER 1

THE PUERTO RICANS

THE HISPANIC POPULATION OF THE UNITED STATES

According to the US Census Bureau (Campbell, 1996 p. 2),

> the Hispanic origin population is projected to increase rapidly over the
> 1995 to 2025 projection period, accounting for 44 percent of the growth in
> the Nation's population (32 million Hispanics out of a total of 72 million
> persons added to the Nation's population).

Even with the likely impact that this anticipated increase in the Hispanic
population should have on the United States, not much effort has been
made to better know these groups of peoples who are often lumped
together in research studies simply as Hispanics.

As of March 1999, the US Census estimates that 70% of the 31.7
million Hispanics reside in four states: California, Texas, New York, and
Florida. The distribution of Hispanics in the United States reported in the
March 1999 *Current Population Survey* (Ramirez, 2000) was Mexican
(65.2%), Central and South American (14.3%), Puerto Rican (9.6%),
Cuban (4.3%), and other Hispanic (6.6%).

Certain common characteristics based on a common heritage are
found among the many Hispanic groups in the United States:

All the groups share a common colonial founding and experience with Spain, and all geographic areas of Latin America witnessed a subjugation, or virtual elimination, of a native population. The native presence remains strong in many, though not all, parts of Latin America...Many parts of Latin America also experienced the introduction of African slavery...Similarly, all countries of Latin America developed an uneasy relationship with the United States reaching back centuries, and the friction between an essentially Mediterranean culture with an Anglo-Saxon one continues to this day...

Although harder to define, there are also many common cultural reflexes that originated in the Iberian Peninsula. The stress on the importance of a large, extended family, the cultivation of personal relationships and alliances, definitions of honor and respect, the distrust of government in general, stratifications based on class and occupation and the adherence, generally, to the same religious identification all stem from Spain. (Rodriguez, 1995 p. 6)

Notwithstanding the similarities, each Hispanic group has its own distinctiveness. Rodriquez attributed the cultural distinctiveness to factors such as: (1) the strength of the native populations that were in the area when the Spaniards and other colonizers arrived that determined whether they were totally eliminated by the mistreatments suffered; (2) the specific distinctive areas (Northern Spain, Canary Islands, Majorca, etc.) from where the Spaniards originated; and (3) differences in the level of introduction of Africans through slavery (mainly in the Caribbean).

Linda Robinson (1998) of *U S News & World Report* has succinctly reported on and classified the Hispanic populations that are found in a wide variety of areas of the United States. (Much of the following description is based on this report.) Hispanic populations are found in a wide variety of areas of the United States. The largest population of individuals of Mexican descent is found in California, Texas, Arizona, New Mexico, and Colorado. Nevertheless, jobs at the steel mills during Word War II attracted a sizable Mexican community to Chicago, which still remains. In addition to differences regarding region where they live,

Mexican Americans have subgroups based on their ancestral ties to North America. That is, Tejanos (Texans of Mexican ancestry) have been in the land for many generations and some families were on this land before the Anglos arrived, while in California the majority of Mexicans reflect a more "recent" arrival from all regions of Mexico.

Central and South Americans in the United States consist mainly of Guatemalans, Nicaraguans, and Colombians. These groups have arrived in the United States since the 1980s when their countries were suffering economic and political unrest. The largest of the Guatemalan groups, mainly Mayan, is found in Houston, Texas, where it has built its own community and successfully joined the working classes. Nicaraguans who arrived in the Miami area have not been so fortunate. According to *US News & World Report*, they "...were embraced by Cubans who sympathized with their flight from communism" (Robinson, 1998, p. 5) and were provided with jobs in Cuban-owned businesses. However, their lack of English skills and education in general keeps them as one of the poorest groups in the area. Colombians, located mainly in Miami and New York City, have reached economic success in this country as business people. Nevertheless, the stereotype of Colombians as drug dealers has been thought to be detrimental to the group's image despite their successes in legitimate enterprises.

Puerto Ricans have migrated to this country since the Spanish American War of 1898 and currently are found throughout the East Coast of the United States, from South Florida to Boston, Massachusetts. In addition, Chicago has attracted a sizable Puerto Rican community. Unlike other Hispanic groups, Puerto Ricans are born American citizens (a right they have had since 1917), but this status has not had the positive impact one might assume, since Puerto Ricans have the highest poverty rates and highest levels of unemployment and female heads of household of any Hispanic group (United States Census Bureau, 1999).

Cubans have migrated to this country, to Ybor City (Tampa) and New York City, since the turn of the 19th century. However, it was the influx of Cubans arriving in the Miami area, New York, and northern New Jersey as they left Cuba fleeing from Fidel Castro's communist government that can be seen as defining the Cuban community in the United States today. This latter wave arrived in the United States in the 1960s and continues in much smaller numbers to the present. The first wave consisted largely of middle- and upper-class professionals who were able to succeed at a faster pace than any other Hispanic group and provide opportunities to the less affluent Cubans who followed.

Among the groups categorized by the Census as "other Hispanics" includes Dominicans, Hondurans, Peruvians, and Salvadorians. These groups also are increasing in number throughout the United States with different levels of success.

The three largest Hispanic groups—Mexicans, Puerto Ricans, and Cubans—share some cultural traits, mainly centering around the use of the Spanish language, but not a common history or set of cultural values. The Cuban exile ethos creates an obviously different mind-set from the Puerto Rican who moves freely to and from "the Island" (as Puerto Ricans often call Puerto Rico) and feels political and social identification with both nations. The Mexicans in the United States may be further categorized into three broad categories: the Californians, the Tejanos (of Texas), and the Chicagoans. Each group is further divided into the newcomers with stronger ties to Mexico and the middle class who usually have been here a generation or more.

Because of the inclusions of respondents from the many different Hispanic groups, problems of labeling and sampling are created for researchers, leading to difficulties of interpretation of research literature. Despite some movement for clarification in governmental studies, e.g., census data, there still is a tendency in much of the literature, especially in nongovernmental national samples, for researchers to label all persons of Mexican, Puerto Rican, Cuban, Central and South American backgrounds as well as those from Spain "Hispanic."

THE PUERTO RICANS IN NEW YORK

An assessment of the Puerto Rican community in New York City compiled by the city's Department of City Planning provides one of the best pictures of that 1989 community in New York at the time the data used in this study were collected. According to the *Puerto Rican New Yorkers in 1990* (Salvo, Ortiz, & Lobo, 1994), Puerto Ricans constituted one of the largest ethnic groups in the city (12% of the population). Nevertheless, this report based mainly on the 1980 and 1990 census data also indicated that "...during the 1970s and 1980s, Puerto Rican out-migrants exceeded Puerto Rican in-migrants" (p. 109). For the years 1985–1990, out-migrants from New York City exceeded in-migrants by 141,595 to 51,526 for persons aged 5 and older. The destination for the largest group of those leaving New York City was found to be "the Island" (38.4%), followed by "elsewhere in New York and New Jersey" (26.4%), and Florida (14.1%). The likelihood for the change in migration patterns may be due to the lack of industrial and blue-collar jobs in the New York City area, as well as the aging of those who came to the mainland in the 1940s and 1950s, who are retiring and returning to Puerto Rico.

Salvo et al. (1994) found that Puerto Ricans in New York City were younger than the general population (median age of 28 vs. 35), but were showing some aging from the 1980 census where the median age among Puerto Ricans was 24. A possible impact of the aging of the Puerto Rican community was found in the decrease in fertility levels. Fertility levels, as measured by the child–women ratio, although still higher than the general population, had dramatically declined from a ratio of 502 children under the age of 5 per 1000 women in 1970 to 395 in 1980 and 359 in 1990.

According to *Puerto Rican New Yorkers in 1990*, "for the first time, a clear majority of Puerto Rican New Yorkers were born in the 50 states" (Salvo et al., 1994, p. 17), reflecting the impact of previous migration years by Puerto Ricans to the mainland United States. The high birthrate of Puerto Rican children in New York City may be viewed with some alarm when considering the household and family compositions of Puerto Ricans in New York City. The report states that "...as a proportion of total households, Puerto Ricans have dramatically more female-head of families and fewer married couples, relative to the general population" (Salvo et al., 1994, p. ii). Nevertheless, by 1990, a decline in this trend was found, but "...while the number of female-headed families with own children actually declined by 10% between 1980 and 1990, the number of female-headed families with no own children increased by 81 percent in this period" (Salvo et al., 1994, p. 26). The aging of the Puerto Rican community, resulting in a less fertile population as well as a higher rate of separated or divorced persons, helps explain these changes in the 1990s.

Although there had been an increase of Puerto Ricans aged 25 and above who had achieved high school diplomas, from 35% in 1980 to 46% in 1990, this was still much lower than the general population (69%). The disparity between Puerto Ricans and the general population was even greater for those who had graduated from college (6% of Puerto Ricans vs. 23% in the general population). Perhaps as a result of lower education levels, the percentage "...of Puerto Rican family income to that of all families remains at 56 percent" despite the 30% increase in real income found between the 1970s and the 1990s (Salvo et al., 1994, p. iii).

A somewhat encouraging finding was made regarding the positive impact of more education on Puerto Rican participation in the labor force. The *Puerto Rican New Yorkers 1990* finds that, "...for male and female Puerto Ricans, as education increases, labor force participation rates converge with those for city residents" (Salvo et al., 1994, p. 72). The changing economic picture of New York City and the United States in general (from a manufacturing to a more service-oriented economy) also has obviously affected Puerto Ricans. The Puerto Rican "representation in *managerial* and *professional* occupations was still low in

1990....(However) the heavy reliance on unskilled and semi-skilled
manufacturing jobs, the historical hallmark of Puerto Rican employment,
is no longer apparent (pp. iii, iv).

AN EMERGING ALCOHOL AND SUBSTANCE ABUSE PROBLEM

The changing and often undesirable economic and social conditions
of the population of Puerto Ricans in New York City have been
accompanied by the frustrations and stress that change often brings. By
the 1960s, concern with the rise in all forms of substance abuse was
increasing throughout the United States. The Puerto Rican community in
New York was not immune from these problems. On an optimistic note,
there was a widespread belief that problematic substance use, misuse,
abuse, and addiction were primarily the products of so-called "slum"
communities in such cities as New York. As reassurance, many service
providers, looked to the island of Puerto Rico itself and some middle-
class communities in Denver, among other cities, as being essentially
drug free and suitable for relocating patients to relatives who lived there.
During the 1960s, one of the authors of this volume worked at several of
the drug and alcoholism treatment centers in East Harlem, the
metropolitan New York neighborhood comprising mainly Puerto Rican
and other Caribbean Hispanics.   One of the available adjuncts to
treatment after detoxification was to send Puerto Rican drug addicts and
alcoholics down to family members in Puerto Rico to get them away
from the substance abuse scene in New York because these problems
seemed almost absent on "the Island."

There was a widely held belief among treatment providers in the
East Harlem community that the traditionally low alcoholism and
substance abuse rates, and in particular the low alcohol use rates of
women on the island of Puerto Rico prior to the 1970s, was rapidly
changing for the worse here on the mainland. Despite the efforts of the
social services and helping professions, an increase in alcohol and drug

problems among the Hispanic populations of New York City was apparent. By the 1980s there was a realization that the problem was widespread but there was no scientific study that detailed the patterns of alcohol and drug use and how these patterns are related to changes in the social world of Hispanics such as acculturation, loss of tradition, employment, education, time in the United States, religion, fatalism, and other social influences outside of the Mexican American community, which had received some scientific study.

In the late 1980s the Hispanic Research Center at Fordham University in New York City was aware that although there was some literature on drug use among Puerto Ricans in New York that included some references to alcohol problems, there was no systematic study of alcohol use patterns themselves among mainland Puerto Ricans. A study was designed to fill this lacuna that could also relate drug use to the same factors that might be influencing alcohol patterns.

AIMS AND SCOPE OF STUDY

The general aims of the researchers at the Fordham Hispanic Research Center, under the direction of Dr. Gerald Gurin, were to collect data on the drinking patterns, drinking attitudes, and gender norms of Puerto Ricans, along with information on alcohol-related problems and how they were coped with by drinkers, family and friends. The Hispanic Research Center intended to obtain information in a manner comparable to that collected by the Berkeley Alcohol Research Center, among other researchers, of Mexican Americans, Anglos, and blacks. A third major aim was to provide information on cultural determinants that could be used in the creation of programs that would be geared more specifically to this population. A need for a study of this type among Puerto Ricans, the dominant Hispanic group in New York, was demonstrated by the fact that the state of New York in 1983 had few reliable data on Hispanic drinking except for a 1969 alcoholism prevalence report (Cahalan, Cisin,

& Crossley, 1969) in order to develop policy regarding alcoholism that was relevant to the Hispanic population. It should be noted that the Cahalan study was conducted using national data that included only 2% Latin Americans or those of Caribbean descent.

The data collected by the Fordham Hispanic Research Center are unique among studies in the eastern United States because it was designed to focus only on Hispanics, specifically Puerto Ricans. Thus, it would provide a large enough sample, unlike other surveys, which would allow for analyses beyond descriptive statistics. The questionnaire took into consideration prevalent assumptions in the field as well as research findings that were specific to Hispanic alcohol use and abuse. One objective was to measure such assumptions as Hispanics being "particularly at risk for alcohol related problems…but they receive less help with these problems from formal treatment sources (than other groups, ed.)" (Gurin, 1986, p. 23)   In addition, differences based on gender found in studies among other Hispanic groups were addressed. These focused on the commonly held views, as well as research findings mainly among Mexican Americans, that the Hispanic culture is "unusually supportive of drinking for Hispanic men and unusually restrictive of drinking for Hispanic women" (Gurin, 1986, p. 24); that Hispanic men drink more than non-Hispanic US whites, but Hispanic women drink less than US whites, regardless of gender; and that the cultural meaning of alcohol use (attitudes, expectations, norms) differs for males and females. The study also included questions that would allow analyses on the impacts that age, education, social class, and generation in the United States have on drinking patterns and problems.

While the study was to include the data to measure acculturation, it also was to include sufficient data to study traditional gender norms to provide measurement for their impact on alcohol use and abuse and to a lesser degree other substance abuse.

DATA AND METHODOLOGY

The data used in this study were collected under a Department of Health and Human Services grant given to the Hispanic Research Center at Fordham University in New York City. The purpose of the grant was to conduct a cross–sectional survey of drinking behavior and norms among Puerto Rican adults.

The data consist of a representative sample taken from the general population of Puerto Ricans living in the New York City metropolitan area. For the study and throughout this volume a Puerto Rican is defined as any person who was born in Puerto Rico, or any person for whom at least one parent or grandparent was born in Puerto Rico and who identified herself or himself as a Puerto Rican.

The Hispanic Research Center subcontracted the task of actual data collection to the Institute for Survey Research (ISR) at Temple University in Philadelphia. The sampling design used was a multistage disproportionate stratified area probability sample. At the first stage, block groups in 10 counties of the greater New York metropolitan area were stratified by county and concentration of Puerto Rican residents. The counties included Bronx, Kings, Nassau, New York, Queens, Richmond, and Suffolk in New York state, as well as Passaic, Essex, and Hudson counties in New Jersey. At the second stage, 300 block groups were selected disproportionately across areas that had a concentration of 10% or more of Puerto Ricans according to the census counts. Higher concentration Puerto Rican strata were oversampled to increase screening efficiency. The sample of household units was selected from listing areas consisting of one to three blocks within the group blocks.

Interviewers screened all households in the sample, obtaining information on the residents' age, gender, and whether or not they were Puerto Rican. Whenever there was more than one eligible resident in a household, only one was randomly selected. A total of 1084 interviews were conducted, 446 males and 638 females, between March 1988 and

March 1989. Respondents were paid $10.00 as an incentive to participate in the study.

These data are needed to fill existing gaps in the literature primarily dealing with alcohol use and to a lesser degree other substances among Hispanics, specifically those of Puerto Rican descent. These gaps are often caused by the small size of the Hispanic sample in existing studies as well as a lack of inquiry into and examination of cultural factors and how they relate to drinking and drug use practices. Although existing general population studies contain data on Hispanic alcohol and other substance use patterns, these studies include too few Hispanics to allow for in-depth statistical controls or for reliable multivariate analyses. The small samples have usually limited the analyses to simple prevalence comparisons between groups, such as Hispanic use versus whites and/or blacks.

The limitation placed on the examination of the data by these small samples is not restricted to findings among different ethnic groups, but also has constricted the analyses possible within the different Hispanic subgroups. Although some studies indicate that there are differences in drinking and drug use patterns and consequences between Hispanic males and females and other studies have found that factors such as education tends to affect the level of drinking in which females engage, the relatively small sizes of the Hispanic samples in these studies have been insufficient to examine these relationships in depth.

Another gap the data presented in this volume attempt to close is the absence of data regarding how traditional norms and attitudes influence drinking and drug use in a specific Hispanic population: in this case, Puerto Ricans. Although existing studies provide prevalence estimates on substance use, they tend to be limited in their scope of cultural and attitudinal factors related to alcohol and drug use. The present study contains areas that are comparable to those studied by the Alcohol Research Group in Berkeley, California, mainly among Hispanics of Mexican origin. Among the areas covered in the Berkeley as well as in this study are drinking consumption, drinking-related problems, drinking in the context of family and work life, attitudes and traditional norms regarding drinking, responses to drinking problems, attitudes toward treatment and treatment experience, and an acculturation scale. Therefore, these data, when compared with the Berkeley data, will provide information to fill in many of the existing gaps that exist in the literature regarding comparisons of two Hispanic groups—Mexican and Puerto Rican. The samples of both are large enough to allow for descriptive information that can be generalizable to each of the two Hispanic populations and allow examination of different demographic subgroups and multivariate analyses of the data.

A unique contribution of this study is that by concentrating on Puerto Ricans there is a large enough sample to allow for the exploration of findings relating to different demographic subgroups within the mainland Puerto Rican population and how these different subgroups are affected by the Puerto Rican culture while the respondents are in mainland United States. By focusing on cultural norms and related behaviors and how these may influence drinking patterns, these data go well beyond other studies of Hispanic populations which allows for a formal examination of conjectures presented by other researchers in the field of Hispanic alcohol use but which have not been measured before. In addition, by providing measures of levels of acculturation, these data provide the opportunity to examine the impact that moving to the United States may have on the cultural norms themselves that may in turn affect drinking and other substance use.

DESCRIPTION OF THE SAMPLE

Interviews were conducted with 1084 adults: 638 females and 446 males. (Due to the often strong cultural differences between men and women regarding norms and values related to substance use, we will often present and analyze data by gender.) The respondents ranged in age from 18 to 87, with a median age of 40.5 for the males and 38.0 for the females. Over a third (37.9%) were married or cohabiting, less than a third (29.1%) were separated or divorced, 7.1% widowed and 25.9% "never married." We present these marital status self-designation findings with a caveat. Data on marital status is tenuous in many studies, since alternative lifestyles have become so common in the United States. A person who has never married may live with a number of partners in serial monogamous relationships, but at the time of the interview be in between relationships and thus specify "single," while another person who may have been abandoned by a spouse might still legitimately say that they are "married." Similarly, a divorced person who is now living in a stable relationship with someone may correctly cite either "divorced" or "cohabiting." Our experience with previous studies has shown the difficulty of not only this classification (in the absence of a long cumbersome list of alternatives) but several others such as "race," "ethnicity," "religion," and "occupation."

Nearly three quarters of the sample (71.1%) were born in Puerto Rico (closely divided between the sexes: 70% of males and 72% of females) while 28.1% were born in mainland United States. A few (8) were born elsewhere. For the 768 persons not born in mainland United States, the average age at time of arrival to the mainland was 20.0 years. The mean for females was 19.9 and the median 19.0. Similarly, for males the mean was 20.2 and the median 19.0.

Nearly half (45.2%) the sample who were born in Puerto Rico were raised for most of their first 16 years in medium-sized cities (25,000 or smaller), while 27.2% were raised in rural communities or farms and an additional 27.6% in the larger cities. Most still declare themselves to be Catholic (80.5%), while an additional 12.5% say they are Protestant.

The level of education, among other sociodemographics, has been cited as one of the most important variables correlated with or predicting levels of acculturation for Puerto Ricans living in the United States (Cuadrado, 1997; Kranau, Green, & Valencia-Weber, 1982; Ready, 1991;

Soto, 1983). As Table 1.1 shows, a majority of adult Puerto Ricans in our sample were dropouts in high school or at even lower grades. Females were slightly more likely to drop out than males (65.0% vs. 59.1%).

As noted in a New York City Planning Department report on the demographic, social, and economic status of Puerto Ricans:

Although there were modest improvements in the 1960s and 1970s, the overall level of educational attainment among Puerto Ricans remained below the national average. Moreover, high school dropout rates among Puerto Ricans have historically been among the highest of any racial or ethnic group." (Salvo et al., 1994, p. 39)

In a footnote, the authors offer a possible explanation for this:

Circular migration has been used to explain the lack of educational success among Puerto Ricans (Fitzpatrick, 1987). The continued back-and-forth migration of Puerto Ricans between the mainland and Puerto Rico has a disruptive effect on the educational process of young Puerto Ricans. This

TABLE 1.1.   Years of Schooling Completed by Gender

Education	Male N	Male %	Female N	Female %	Total N	Total %
None – 4th grade	60	13.5	76	11.9	136	12.6
5th – 8th grade	86	19.3	132	20.7	218	20.1
9th – 11th grade	117	26.3	206	32.4	323	30.0
High school graduate	121	27.2	150	23.5	271	25.0
Some college	50	11.2	63	9.9	113	10.4
College graduate	11	2.5	10	1.6	21	1.9
Total	445*	100.0	637*	100.0	1082	100.0

$\chi^2(5, N = 1082) = 6.91, p > .05$.
* The total samples consisted of 446 males and 638 females.

circular migration is tied to the restructuring of the economy which has limited employment opportunities of Puerto Rican workers both in the Northeast and in Puerto Rico. (p. 44, fn)

Essential to future group mobility and economic success is the educational mobility of a newer immigrant population. Because of the complexity of current technological and service-oriented sectors of the economy, the necessity for higher education for an ever-increasing percentage of the Hispanic populations is crucial. Do Puerto Ricans, as have many other immigrant groups, take advantage of the many educational opportunities in Puerto Rico and mainland United States so that children receive more formal schooling than their parents? In this respect, our findings are dismal (See Table 1.2).

For those respondents whose parents had no college, we find only 12.2% of the offspring with some college. Perhaps more unsettling is the finding that among those respondents having at least one parent with some college or above, less than a third (30.8%) of the children had gone beyond high school. Evidently, the college experience of a parent does not appear to be sufficient to ensure being college bound in the

TABLE 1.2 Comparison of Parental College Education by Respondent College Education

	Parents			
			Total	
Respondent	No college	Mother and/or Father with Some college +	N	%
No college	87.8%	69.2%	756	86.8
Some college +	12.2%	30.8%	115	13.2
N	819	52	871	
Parent's Total %	94.0	6.0	100.0	

χ^2 (1, N = 1082) = 14.58, p < .001.

succeeding generation. It is possible that some in this adult population may elect to go to college later, but certainly not approaching the national averages. One bright spot was the finding that more than twice as many children (13.2%) as their parents (6.0%) have had at least some college.

Over two fifths of the sample (45.7%) were working full or part time at the time of interview. This, of course, is not an accurate representation of the percentage of Puerto Rican families whose income is derived from employment, since other members of the household may be providing an income for those respondents who were not employed (see Table 1.3). Indeed, an additional 156 of the respondents cited others (mother, father, spouse, child, sibling, and others) as providing an income if they did not claim so for themselves. Thus, a total of 650 respondents (60.1%) reporting this information were living in households with at least some income from earnings. While data were not collected on whether or not the household of the respondent was receiving public assistance, the New York City Planning Department reported that this was the case for 35.6% of the Puerto Rican Families in the city (Salvo et al., 1994, p. 60). They also report that the median household income for Puerto Rican households in 1989 was $17,400.

TABLE 1.3. Employment Status by Gender

Employment	Male		Female		Total	
	N	%	N	%	N	%
Employed	310	70.0	184	28.9	494	45.7
Unemployed	54	12.2	33	5.2	87	8.1
In school	15	3.4	26	4.1	41	3.8
Retired	63	14.2	66	10.4	129	11.9
Homemaker	1	0.2	328	51.4	329	30.5
Totals	443	100.0	637	100.0	1080	100.0

$\chi^2(4, N = 1080) = 341.41, p < .001.$

COMING TO THE MAINLAND AND THE ACCULTURATION PROCESS

Why do individuals and families migrate from "the Island" to the mainland? Were their aspirations met? How extensive are their ties to the Island culture? How "Anglocized" have they become? How much English do they speak, read, and write? Do they socialize with non-Hispanics? Do they watch Hispanic TV and listen to Hispanic music? What do they consider their main identity to be: Puerto Rican or American? How do we measure and what is their degree of acculturation and identity?

FROM THE ISLAND TO THE MAINLAND

Of the 1084 Puerto Ricans in the sample, 71% were born in Puerto Rico, closely divided between the sexes (see Chapter 1). Fifty-nine percent of the Puerto Rican women and 64% of the men came to the mainland United States between the years 1950 and 1969. This was the post-World War II era when the United States was expanding its industrial base and was perceived in Puerto Rico as a likely place for individuals to prosper (Passalacqua, 1994; Wargacki, 1986).

The predominant reason given by the respondents in the sample (including those born here) for their family's move from Puerto Rico to the United States was the search for a "better life," reported by 68.3% of the sample (see Table 2.1). Examination of this variable by gender of the respondent showed that men were somewhat more likely than women to cite "better life" (73.0% vs. 64.9%). This probably reflects the male's greater responsibility for earning a living within the Puerto Rican family.

Were their dreams realized? For the most part, yes, as shown by the finding that 77% of the respondents (men and women in almost equal percentages) stated that their family's main objectives were completely or mostly fulfilled. On average these satisfied Puerto Ricans had spent 24.1 years in the United States providing the opportunity for successful fulfillment of their dreams, in particular through their children. This finding is similar to that made by Rogler and Santana (1994) in their

TABLE 2.1. Reason Respondent's Family Moved to the United States by Gender

Why did family move to the United States?	Male		Female		Total	
	N	%	N	%	N	%
Better life	324	73.0	413	64.9	737	68.3
Family/friends in US	101	22.7	190	29.9	291	26.9
Other	19	4.3	33	5.2	52	4.8
Total	444	100.0	636	100.0	1080	100.0

$\chi^2(2, N = 1080) = 7.85, p < .05.$

study of Puerto Ricans migrating to the United States when they conclude: "The hopes and aspirations which led the persons in the parent generation to migrate to New York City are much more fully realized in their offspring" (p. 218).

The ties to "the Island" among mainland Puerto Ricans still remain strong, although the average number of years in the United States was 27.9 with little difference between males and females. Ninety-four percent of the respondents have family or friends in Puerto Rico. Nearly 84% have traveled to Puerto Rico and slightly under half (49.1%) stated they would like to live on "the Island." Almost half (45.1%) stated that they had most of their family in Puerto Rico.

When presented with a list of choices and asked to specify their ethnic identification, almost half (48.4%) of the respondents identified themselves as "all Puerto Rican"; followed by 36.2% who viewed themselves as a combination of "Puerto Rican and American" (see Table 2.2). Women were more likely than men to view themselves as "all Puerto Rican" or "mostly Puerto Rican" (61.2% vs. 52.2%).

TABLE 2.2. Ethnic Self-identification by Gender

Ethnic Identification	Male		Female		Total	
	N	%	N	%	N	%
All Puerto Rican	198	44.6	326	51.2	524	48.4
Mostly Puerto Rican	34	7.6	64	10.0	98	9.0
Puerto Rican and American	179	40.2	213	33.4	392	36.2
Neither Puerto Rican or American	5	1.1	6	0.9	11	1.0
Mostly American	18	4.0	22	3.4	40	3.7
All American	11	2.5	7	1.1	18	1.7
Total	445	100.0	638	100.0	1083	100.0

$\chi^2(5, N = 1083) = 10.73, p > .05.$

Puerto Ricans, unlike other Hispanic groups that have come to the United States, are American citizens from birth; however, almost half the respondents do not identify themselves as Americans and slightly over one third identify themselves as both Puerto Rican and American. It appears that although Puerto Ricans have the status of US citizenship, their identity as Americans may be weaker than that of other so-called hyphenated Americans. The fact that nearly half the sample considers itself "all Puerto Rican" may reflect the Puerto Rican nationalist goals of independence embodied in a cultural desire, held even by the antinationalists, to retain as much of their cultural traits and mores as possible in this perceived "sea of Anglos." Puerto Ricans, as with other immigrant groups, have this strong sense of "we–they"; but unlike other non-Hispanic immigrant cultures, the "we" is magnified and reinforced by the many other Latin groups that are visible on the American scene and their success *as Latinos* in the United States. This is particularly true for the Dominican, Mexican, and Cuban communities that have produced singers, musicians, actors, baseball stars, and others who identify themselves and are identified in the media with their ethnic origins. The images of Sosa, Selena, Estefan, Moreno, Martin, Smits, Santana, and many others are identified positively with their ethnic origins. This is a departure from an earlier generation of Hispanics as well as other ethnic groups in the past who tried to minimize their "differences" from the Anglo culture at a time when their ethnic origins were more likely to become associated in the media with negative stereotypes and images: wetback, peddler, gangster, slaughterhouse worker, among others, buttressed by such derogatory terms as lazy, violent, loud, pushy, dirty, and so on. While this is not to suggest that there is total acceptance of Hispanic groups (or for that matter any immigrant group that is not identified with the Anglo-Saxon core culture), there certainly has been much progress in the latter half of the 20th Century. However, the passion and strength of Latino identification cannot help but be influenced by a continuous period of intolerance toward all Hispanic groups. This is especially true for the Mexican American community, which has had a long history of being the recipients of hostile American-Anglo reactions.

The transition of Puerto Rican men and women to the mainland, as with all immigrant groups, necessitates the learning of a new culture with its language, food, music, rules, customs, and the full range of cultural norms that enables participants in the Anglo society to adequately function. The degree of learning and assimilating these new mores has been termed "acculturation." However, because of the strength of the Puerto Rican culture in the mainland itself, the process of acculturation applies not only to the newcomers but also to those born on the mainland who may have grown up with a narrowing of their social and cultural interactions largely focused within the Hispanic communities. To understand the process of change as it applies to Puerto Ricans and to shed light on the relationship of cultural change to deviant behaviors, the concept of acculturation must be examined more closely.

THE ACCULTURATION PROCESS

Acculturation has been the focus of study in several academic fields. Psychologists in their study of individuals also have used the concept, originally developed by anthropologists and sociologists for studies of groups. Therefore, it is not surprising that Padilla (1980, p. 1) refers to acculturation as an "ambiguous term." Regardless of the focus (group or individual), the definition of acculturation has certain components that have been dissected by Berry (1980), who argued that:

Acculturation requires the contact of at least two autonomous cultural groups; there must also be change in one or other of the two groups which results from the contact....[I]n practice one group dominates the other and contributes more to the flow of the cultural elements than does the weaker of the groups....[Furthermore, t]he apparent domination of one group over the other suggests that what happens between contact and change may be difficult, reactive and conflicting rather than a smooth transition. (p. 10)

Berry (1980, p. 12) goes on to indicate that in addition to contact and conflict, the process of acculturation also is marked by adaptation. Adaptation may be in the form of adjustment ("changes are made which reduce the conflict by making cultural or behavioral features more similar"), reaction ("changes are made which attempt to reduce conflict by retaliating against the source of conflict"), and withdrawal ("changes are made which essentially remove one element from the contact arena"). All three forms of adaptation are readily observable in the Puerto Rican as well as other Hispanic populations residing in the mainland.

For individuals coping with a new culture through Berry's first mode of adaptation (adjustment), the structure of norms that may have guided them through their daily choices in social behavior is no longer valid or at least no longer compelling. As an illustration, a Puerto Rican married woman on the mainland has more freedom to interact with males in a business relationship outside the home. She may attend a staff meeting running late into the evening and have drinks at lunch with a male co-worker. This "adjustment" is often born of the necessity for two income families in the United States.

If adaptation through adjustment becomes the dominant mode of adaptation to the elimination of reaction and withdrawal, the end result will be the loss of those identifying and unique characteristics of this (or any other) immigrant culture in favor of those of the host (Anglo) culture. When this occurs, individuals are said to have been assimilated into the mainstream culture and are virtually indistinguishable from those in the dominant (Anglo) group. This process of assimilation in varying degrees has occurred in most previous immigrant groups, e.g., Poles, Irish, Italians, Eastern Europeans, and so forth, who may on occasion reassert the remnants of their ethnic identity by parades, holidays, dances, food, and so on, but taken as a whole, the sum of daily activities, language spoken, musical tastes, dance styles, everyday cuisine, clothing, manners, and morals are mainstream "American."

This may be contrasted with the development of Puerto Rican youth gangs in East Harlem during the 1960s and 1970s as defense against the hostility of other ethnic youth groups on whose territory they were thought to be impinging: an example of adaptation through *reaction* rather than adjustment.

Withdrawal is probably the most commonly found means of adaptation among mainland Puerto Ricans, e.g., the development of Puerto Rican *bodegas* to carry the desired foods, Puerto Rican music stores, newspapers, and so forth. Some immigrant and ethnic groups have become acculturated to the extent that they can function in the economic and civil aspects of American life but have resisted acculturation that threatens the way of life brought to this country. These are mainly groups strongly tied to highly traditional religious views, e.g., the Amish communities and the Hassidic Jews, perhaps the clearest examples of Berry's "withdrawal" as adaptation.

Clearly, we find a much larger proportion of Hispanic persons—Mexicans, Dominicans, Cubans, Puerto Ricans, and others—among those whose lifestyle could be classified as falling into the "withdrawal" category than those in previous immigrant groups. A unique feature of their situation, having both positive and negative consequences and a source of some controversy, is that the cohesive factor is not tied to a religious identity but rather the desire to retain a linguistic identity in everyday life and other aspects of the culture associated with it: music, dance, food, holidays, and to a lesser degree "interpersonal relations." This has been puzzling to a mainstream America that had absorbed food, music, colloquialisms, and even holidays from many other earlier groups but which was not prepared to accept language differences. The apparent clash of the acculturation process and retention of Hispanic linguistic identity has created significant conflict and mistrust among segments of both the Anglo and

Hispanic communities. Many Puerto Ricans, as do other Hispanic groups, see various "English only" movements as having a hidden agenda to eventually force their assimilation into the Anglo culture.

CULTURAL MARGINALITY

Persons who through migration, education, marriage, or other influences leave their social group or culture of origin without making a satisfactory adjustment to their new group or culture find themselves on the *margin* of each but a member of neither (Stonequist, 1937, p. 3). Immigrants from foreign shores and others who may be moving from one cultural area or group within this country usually find themselves in a social situation reflecting a decrease in the influence of their original culture norms. They are pulled by the different and even antagonistic ways of the new culture in which they now find themselves. These persons have been conceptualized by Stonequist as "marginal men." If individuals lose their attachments to the norms of their original group but have not fully acquired the norms of the group to which they aspire, they may find themselves having difficulty in making appropriate choices (Park & Miller, 1921; Schutz, 1944; Sellin, 1938; Stonequist, 1937).

During the transitional period of adapting to a new culture the controls imposed on individuals by their culture of origin regarding acceptable behavior may weaken due to the waning influence of existing traditional community consensus and sanctions. At the same time, individuals have not yet fully incorporated the controlling norms and values of the host culture, making them more susceptible to engaging in deviant and/or criminal behavior.

This influence of the culture within which one has been raised to limit as well as give permission may conflict with the norms of the host culture. This is certainly the case with alcohol use for many groups. Park and Miller (1921) described the conflict produced on the individual level by this aspect of acculturation as follows:

At home the immigrant was almost completely controlled by the community; in America, this lifelong control is relaxed. Here the community of his people is at best far from complete, and moreover, it is located within the American community, which lives by different and more individualistic standards, and show, as we have seen, a contempt for all the characteristics of the newcomer. All the old habits of the immigrants consequently tend to break down. The new situation has the nature of a crisis, and in a crisis the individual tends either to reorganize his life positively, or to repudiate the old habits and their restraints without reorganizing his life—which is demoralization. (p. 61)

Substance use, both alcohol and illicit drugs, may present a special problem for Hispanic women and to some extent Hispanic men, since Anglo culture provides more freedom regarding drinking in particular but does not provide clear and consistent norms regarding alcohol and drug use for men or women. Puerto Rican women, if raised in a traditional setting, will have clearly defined norms regarding the use of alcohol (which plausibly generalize to the use of other drugs as well) that enforce abstinence. However, in mainland United States, Puerto Rican women have greater freedom to choose to drink, but the clarity of norms regarding substance use (other than the criminal consequences) from peers is not present. The heterogeneous makeup of the population in the United States, with abstinence for some groups, only ceremonial drinking for others, and undefined freedom of social drinking for most including the modern urban woman, does not allow for one set of norms to be present.

A commonly offered explanation for excessive drinking and drug use by Puerto Rican males frequently heard among counselors working with Hispanic problem drinkers and substance abusers is that the cultural norm of *machismo* dictates that men should have the social right and the ability to consume a great deal of alcohol; these counselors report that some males have extended this to include drug use. It has been noted that elements of the culture itself encourage and sanction drinking among men (Panitz, McConchie, Sauber, & Fonseca, 1983; Vazquez-Nuttall, Avila-Vivas, & Morales-Barreto, 1984) and it is conceivable that some men may interpret this permission to apply to drug use as well (Quintero & Estrada, 1998).

Another theorist who has expanded on the concept of the conflict suffered by immigrants is Alfred Schutz (1944). Schutz used the term "stranger" to describe "the adult individual of our times and civilization who tries to be permanently accepted or at least tolerated by the group which he approaches" (p. 499). Schutz views the individual who is born into a culture as being able to act without questioning the coherence or contradictions of that system. Any member born or reared within the group accepts the ready-made scheme of the cultural patterns handed down by ancestors, teachers, and authorities as a guide in all the situations that normally occur within the social world (p. 501). They will have acquired a "knowledge of trustworthy *recipes* for interpreting the social world and for handling things and men in order to obtain the best results in every situation with a minimum of effort" (p. 501). The culture thus provides what Schutz calls "thinking as usual," the "of course" assumptions relevant to a particular group that function to "eliminate troublesome inquires by offering ready-made directions for use, to replace truth hard to obtain with comfortable truism" (p. 501). The task of the stranger who is becoming acculturated is to learn the recipes and "thinking as usual" of the culture he or she may be approaching. This may be more difficult than may appear, for the newcomer will often question and misinterpret the ways of the culture being approached.

The fact of being American citizens before migrating to the mainland may paradoxically inhibit or distort the acculturation process for Puerto Ricans. Since Puerto Ricans can so easily travel between "the Island" and the United States, and they are likely to have family and friends in Puerto Rico, they are repeatedly confronted with the reality of living in both cultures, thus reducing their commitment to the new culture in which they live when they return to the mainland. Furthermore, the existence of a viable Puerto Rican community in mainland United States, as well as the presence of other Hispanic communities, also enables them to maintain the folkways of "the Island" culture and to only minimally embrace the new. This may be particularly problematic for the children of immigrant Puerto Ricans, who according to Diaz and Draguns (1990, p. 36) "may resist the Puerto Rican heritage, [but] they have no roots on the mainland."

Not all view the lack of acculturation as a lack of commitment on the part of Puerto Ricans, but as the result of rejection on the part of Anglos. Passalacqua (1994), for example, discusses findings by a public opinion firm charged with studying the perception of Puerto Ricans in the United States as follows:

> Puerto Rico was seen as poor, unstable and backward. The neighboring island of Jamaica was seen in a more favorable light....Puerto Ricans—said a whopping 40 per cent of Americans—are poor because they are lazy. Among those interviewed, the preferred solution to the relationship was to grant independence to Puerto Rico (33 percent) and the least preferred was to grant statehood (20 percent). (p. 106)

Anglo rejection is likely to have had an impact on Puerto Rican acculturation, but it should be noted that most immigrants are exposed to some level of rejection and discrimination by the host group. This suggests that there are other factors, in addition to Anglo rejection, that more greatly influence Puerto Rican identity and acculturation levels.

Adjusting or acculturating is not always the panacea that many believe it should be for the immigrant coming to this country, since the end of the process may be assimilation. According to Berry (1980), conflict may continue throughout the process of adaptation. Acculturation therefore may be viewed as a process to be measured on a continuum defined by the retention of the original cultural identity and the degree of acceptance of the norms of the dominant group. Thus, different degrees of adaptation (acculturation) will be found among the individuals of the many immigrant groups.

ACCULTURATION AMONG PUERTO RICANS

Literature on how acculturation affects Puerto Ricans in daily life matters is scarce. Nevertheless, some authors have described life for Puerto Ricans on "the Island" and in the mainland United States, offering the possibility of some inferences (Aguirre-Molina, 1991; Diaz & Draguns, 1990; Padilla, 1958; Soto, 1983; Torre, Rodriquez Vecchini, & Burgos, 1994). Most Puerto Ricans come to the United States in search of a better life for themselves and their families. A better life was defined by improved economic opportunities (Padilla, 1958; Rogler & Santana Cooney, 1994). However, few can be aware of or prepared for the impact that moving to a country that is so different from their own will have on their previous way of life.

As with other immigrants, Puerto Ricans who move to the mainland find that adhering to the norms that are part of the Puerto Rican culture may no longer be the comfortable and unquestionable path to follow. They soon learn that there are cultural differences inherent in the Anglo norms that now may create conflict. For example, the notion that a wife must be subordinate to her husband's wishes and lifestyle (i.e., she should maintain the pure and virtuous image that includes not working outside the home and retreating to the background of women in mixed company) conflicts with the greater equality norms of the husband–wife roles in mainland America that have been developing over the last four decades. Puerto Ricans on the mainland (the stranger) find themselves in situations where "thinking as usual" is no longer possible. They can no longer react to situations in the same manner as they would in the traditional family on "the Island."

One important source of problems is employment. Until the relatively full employment of the latter half of the 1990s it was often easier for Puerto Rican women to find employment than it was for their husbands (Ghali, 1982). This gave women a sense of independence they may not have had on "the Island," while at the same time it may have resulted in demeaning the role of the "man of the house." This unexpected role displacement that is imposed on the family by the new environment can be very disruptive of family life as was known back in Puerto Rico. Wives working outside the home may not only demean the role of the man who was raised in the traditional culture, but it also exposes women to attitudes and behaviors that they may not have encountered before, such as casual social drinking by other women—a violation of traditional drinking norms and constraints. Children (who are likely to learn the language better than their parents) may not be spared the confusions affecting traditional adult role relationships, since they are often relied on to serve as interpreters, making their parents and other adults feel even more inadequate and the youngster ashamed for this parental inadequacy (Ghali, 1982). These stresses can be characterized as the breakdown of the "known" way of life, of the specific roles of different members of the family and the norms attached to these roles.

ACCULTURATION AS A FACTOR IN SUBSTANCE USE

When we examine the literature on Hispanics and deviant substance use (both alcohol and illicit drugs), we find that the most common explanation offered for this behavior is the process of acculturation. While many researchers appear to view the acquisition of new values as a valid explanation for substance abuse, others more specifically interpret the consequences of acculturation such as stress, loss of proscriptive norms, better education, and anomie as the main explanatory factors (Alcocer, 1982; Amaro, Coffman, & Herren, 1990; Caetano, 1984a,b, 1986, 1987a,b, 1988; Canino, 1994; Cuadrado & Lieberman, 1998; Farabee, Wallisch, & Maxwell, 1995; Graves, 1967; Madsen, 1964; Markides, Krause, & Mendes de Leon, 1988; Perez, Padilla, Ramirez, Ramirez, & Rodriguez, 1980; Szalay, Canino, & Vilov, 1993; Vega, Alderete, Kolody, & Aguilar-Gaxiola, 1998; Vega, Gil,

Warheit, Zimmerman, & Apospori, 1993; Wagner-Echeagaray, Schutz, Chilcoat, & Anthony, 1994).

A theme that runs through many of the research studies of the acculturation process that may contribute to an understanding of how acculturation influences substance abuse is the degree to which an immigrant has learned and accepted the new norms and values. Social Control theorists have argued that an individual's response to the possibility of engaging in deviant behavior will depend on the strength of his or her bond with the norms and values of society (Hirschi, 1969). These bonds usually are viewed as the norms and values of one's own culture acquired during the early socialization processes or the norms and values of the host culture acquired during the resocialization process, that is, acculturation. This suggests that in the absence of understanding and accepting the new host norms governing behavior, the older traditional norms need to be relied on unless situational factors have loosened their controlling hold on the individual. For such an individual in transition from one culture to another without the necessary controlling norms to guide behavior we may say that he or she is now in a state of *anomie* or "normlessness" with respect to that part of social behavior. This element of "marginality" also has been cited as a source of substance abuse problems among some Hispanics who have reacted to the stresses of marginality by coping mechanisms involving the use of alcohol (Neff, Hoppe, & Parea, 1987).

THE MEASUREMENT OF ACCULTURATION

One of the difficulties with acculturation has been to choose which among the many possible elements of one's lifestyle and demographics should define its usage for statistical research. Must we bring in such influences as which generation in the United States, the level of education, aspirations to be assimilated, daily cuisine, keeping up with the "old country," visits to Puerto Rico or Mexico, or the full range of measures of language, media preference, social interactions, and identity?

The main elements of the measurement of acculturation had been spelled out as early as 1967 by Graves as *"adoption* of certain Anglo-American norms...*exposure* to various middle-class beliefs and values...*Identification* with the dominant society...*access* to the social and material goals of that society" (Graves, 1967, p. 309) rather than what one has given up by way of loss of parts of the culture of origin. This lacuna in measurement of processes in the transition from one culture to another will be addressed in later chapters by examining the consequences of the loss of traditional values.

The complexity of the acculturation concept often has led researchers to attempt to measure it by using multiple variables and in a variety of ways. Nonetheless, certain factors appear to be common: language knowledge and preference and the ethnic background of the people the respondent mingles with in different environments. In this volume, we have used these acculturation items as well as others to create an instrument to measure the degree of acculturation. We modeled this index after the acculturation index developed and validated by Raul Caetano at the Alcohol Research Group at Berkeley (Caetano, 1987a,b).

Among the data collected were 27 variables that could be used to measure acculturation. These variables replicated those used by Caetano at Berkeley. Listed in factor-loading order from highest to lowest, they are:

1. Do you speak mostly English or Spanish with your friends or about the same?
2. Interview conducted in English or Spanish?
3. Do you speak Spanish (if interviewed in English)?
4. Do you speak mostly English or Spanish with your brother/sister or about the same?

5. Do you speak mostly English or Spanish with your husband/spouse (live in) or about the same?

6. Do you speak English (if interviewed in Spanish)?

7. Do you speak mostly English or Spanish with your children or about the same?

8. Do you speak mostly English or Spanish with your neighbors or about the same?

9. Do you speak mostly English or Spanish with the people at work or about the same?

10. When you read a book/magazine/novela do you prefer to read a Spanish language version?

11. Would you say you write English?

12. Would you say you read English?

13. When you listen to the radio do you prefer to listen to Hispanic rather than American stations?

14. When you watch TV do you prefer to watch Hispanic rather than American channels?

15. Do you speak mostly English or Spanish with your other relatives or about the same?

16. When you listen to music do you prefer to listen to Hispanic rather than American music?

17. Do you speak mostly English or Spanish with your parents or about the same?

18. Thinking of the parties you usually go to these days, what proportion of the people there are Hispanics?

19. It is better that Hispanics only marry other Hispanics.

20. Thinking of your friends that you usually see these days, what proportion are Hispanic?

21. Socially, I feel less comfortable with Americans than with Hispanics.

22. When you speak English, do you have a lot of problems, some problems, or no problem in making yourself understood?

23. When you hear English spoken, do you have a lot of problems, some problems, or no problem in understanding what you hear?

24. Would you say you read Spanish very well, well, not very well, or do you not read Spanish?

25. Would you say you write Spanish very well, well, not very well, or do you not write Spanish?

26. Think of the people in the neighborhood where you live now; are they all or nearly all Hispanic, about half Hispanic, less than half Hispanic, few or none Hispanic?

27. Thinking of your current church congregation, what proportion are Hispanic: all or nearly all of them, about half of them, less than half of them, few or none or them, never go to church.

Since Caetano's index was validated with a Mexican American population, the acculturation index developed for this study was revalidated with the Puerto Rican sample. Factor analysis (principal component) was used to determine which of the possible 27 acculturation items should be kept and incorporated into the acculturation scale. All items constituting factor one (items 1–21) were kept. The factor loadings ranged from a high of .86883 for item 1 to a low of .45115 for item 21. Factor one accounted for 44.5% of the variance with an Eigenvalue of 12.02. As suggested by Caetano (1987a), 16 of the 21 variables kept after factor analysis were combined into four indices:

1. Ability to speak English
2. Ability to read and/or write English
3. Use of English with family, friends, and at work
4. Media language preference

The "ability to speak English" index was created by assigning the respondents to one of three categories ("Spanish only," "bilingual" or "English only") according to the language (English or Spanish) used during the interview and whether they spoke the other language (the one not used during the interview). Respondents who were interviewed in Spanish and who said that they did not speak English were assigned to a "Spanish only" category; respondents who were interviewed in Spanish and did speak English, as well as respondents who were interviewed in English but who spoke Spanish were assigned to a "bilingual" category; and respondents who were interviewed in English and who said that they did not speak Spanish were assigned to the "English only" category.

Two questions were asked of respondents in order to rate their ability to read and write English from "very well," assigned a value of 4 (higher score indicating direction of higher acculturation), to "do not read (or write) English," assigned a value of 1. The "ability to read/write English" index was created by adding the responses to these two questions for a maximum score of 8 indicating high ability (and higher acculturation).

The "use of English with family, friends, and at work" index was created by adding the responses to the matrix question "Do you speak mostly Spanish or English with (spouse or partner, children, brother and sister, parents, other relatives, friends, neighbors, and people at work), or do you use both about the same?" Possible responses were "mostly Spanish," with an assigned value of 1; "mostly English," with an assigned value of 3; and "both about the same," with an assigned value of 2. In cases with missing values or in instances where the question did not apply, the average obtained from all other items in the scale was substituted. A maximum score of 24 indicated the highest level of English use with others.

The "media language preference" index consisted of adding the responses to questions regarding whether the respondent preferred to read books and magazines, listen to radio, and watch television in Spanish rather than English. The responses ranged from "most of the time," with a value of 1 to "rarely or never," with a value of 4. A maximum score of 12 indicated the highest preference for English media.

These four indices and the five remaining items ("Socially, I feel less comfortable with Americans than with Hispanics," "It is better that Hispanics only marry other Hispanics," "When listening to music, do you prefer to listen to Hispanic rather than American music," "Thinking of your friends that you usually see these days, what proportion are Hispanic" "Thinking of the parties you usually go to these days, what proportion of these people are Hispanic") were combined to create the acculturation index. The responses to the five items (other than the indices) were scored between 1 and 4 with the higher number indicating higher acculturation. The scores and percent of respondents for each item are presented in Table 2.3.

The responses provided by men to the acculturation index items indicate that they are more highly acculturated than women are. In all but two items, males were more likely to score as more acculturated than females were. Men were more likely to be bilingual or only English speakers, to be able to read and write English, to use English when communicating with others, to prefer American media, to feel socially comfortable with Anglos, to have a higher proportion of Anglo friends, and to prefer American music than were the women. The two items for which there were no significant differences were related to marriage and party going. The finding that Puerto Rican men are more likely to be acculturated than Puerto Rican women probably reflects the more sheltered environments in which women usually live which does not readily expose them to the Anglo culture. Although Puerto Rican women have been found to obtain employment with greater ease than their male counterparts, this does not necessarily mean that the employment is outside of the Hispanic community (Ghali, 1982).

As stated earlier, language is an important indicator of acculturation, often used by researchers as the sole measure. The first three indices reflecting ability to speak, read, and write English have become controversial issues during the last two decades in Puerto Rico and in a

TABLE 2.3. Percent of Respondents by Gender for Each Acculturation
Index Item

	Male		Female		Total	
	N	%	N	%	N	%
1. Index of ability to speak English						
Only Spanish (score 1)	51	11.7	124	20.0	175	16.6
Bilingual (score 2)	373	85.5	486	78.5	859	81.4
Only English (score 3)	12	2.8	9	1.5	21	2.0
Total	436	100.0	619	100.0	1055	100.0

$\chi^2(2, N = 1055) = 14.44, p < .001.$

2. Index of ability to read / write English						
Low (score 2,3)	79	17.8	161	25.3	240	22.2
Med. low (score 4,5)	100	22.5	149	23.4	249	23.0
Med. high (score 6,7)	94	21.2	97	15.2	191	17.7
High (score 8)	171	38.5	230	36.1	401	37.1
Total	444	100.0	637	100.0	1081	100.0

$\chi^2(3, N = 1081) = 12.32, p < .01.$

3. Index of English use with family, friends, and at work						
Low (score 8)	110	24.8	233	37.0	343	32.0
Med. low (score 9–11)	83	18.7	89	14.1	172	16.0
Med. high (score 12–16)	91	20.5	164	26.0	255	23.8
High (score 17–24)	159	36.0	144	22.9	303	28.2
Total	443	100.0	630	100.0	1073	100.0

$\chi^2(3, N = 1073) = 34.41, p < .001.$

4. Index of preference for Hispanic media						
High (score 2,3)	60	13.5	151	23.7	211	19.5
Med. high (score 4,5)	83	18.6	141	22.1	224	20.7
Med. low (score 6–8)	113	25.3	173	27.1	286	26.4
Low (score 9–12)	190	42.6	173	27.1	363	33.4
Total	446	100.0	638	100.0	1084	100.0

$\chi^2(3, N = 1084) = 34.73, p < .001.$

5. Socially less comfortable with Anglos than with Hispanics

Strongly agree (score 1)	53	11.9	123	19.3	176	16.3
Agree (score 2)	103	23.2	165	25.9	268	24.8
Disagree (score 3)	237	53.4	280	44.0	517	47.8
Strongly disagree (score 4)	51	11.5	69	10.8	120	11.1
Total	444	100.0	637	100.0	1081	100.0

$\chi^2(3, N = 1081) = 14.46, p < .01.$

6. Better that Hispanics only marry other Hispanics

Strongly agree (score 1)	4	10.6	87	13.7	134	12.4
Agree (score 2)	112	25.2	158	24.8	270	25.0
Disagree (score 3)	252	56.6	346	54.3	598	55.3
Strongly disagree (score 4)	34	7.6	46	7.2	80	7.4
Total	445	100.0	637	100.0	1082	100.0

$\chi^2(3, N = 1082) = 2.36, p > .05.$

7. Prefer to listen to Hispanic music instead of American

Most or all the time (score 1)	197	44.2	336	52.7	533	49.2
About half (score 2)	124	27.8	197	31.0	321	29.6
Less than half (score 3)	47	10.5	47	7.4	94	8.7
Rarely (score 4)	78	17.5	57	8.9	135	12.5
Total	446	100.0	637	100.0	1083	100.0

$\chi^2(3, N = 1083) = 23.15, p < .001.$

8. Proportion of friends who are Hispanic

All or nearly all (score 1)	295	66.4	482	76.0	777	72.1
About half (score 2)	116	26.1	119	18.8	235	21.8
Less than half (score 3)	18	4.1	21	3.3	39	3.6
Few or none (score 4)	15	3.4	12	1.9	27	2.5
Total	444	100.0	634	100.0	1078	100.0

$\chi^2(3, N = 1078) = 12.51, p < .01.$

9. Proportion of Hispanics at parties

All or nearly all (score 1)	218	65.3	337	72.2	555	69.3
About half (score 2)	80	24.0	102	21.8	182	22.7
Less than half (score 3)	20	6.0	17	3.6	37	4.6
Few or none (score 4)	16	4.7	11	2.4	27	3.4
Total	334	100.0	467	100.0	801	100.0

$\chi^2(3, N = 801) = 7.47, p > .05.$

number of states that have large Hispanic populations. An "English only" sentiment, apparently directed primarily at the Hispanic populations, was reflected in several "official English" pieces of legislation introduced into Congress in the middle 1990s. Although these types of legislation have not passed on the national level, they have had an impact on the Puerto Rican referendum on statehood in 1998. There, opponents of statehood introduced the fears that if Puerto Rico were to become the 51st state, Congress may pass legislation requiring Puerto Rico to conduct official business only in English and require an increase in English language training at the expense of education in Spanish. This was perceived by many as being threatening to their identity as Hispanics by both Puerto Ricans on the island and on the mainland, further strengthening those who wish to see themselves primarily as Puerto Ricans. Nevertheless, the language issue remains a problem, since success and mobility on the mainland for most immigrants are related to their English abilities. As shown in Table 2.3, a large majority (81.4%) of the respondents were bilingual. However, this may be illusory, since there is no clear operational standard for binguality and it may reflect only the informal conversation that the interviewer used to conduct the interview. This is demonstrated by the finding that when we examine item 2 (the self-reported bilingual skills of the respondents) we see that just over one third (37.1%) of the respondents were classified as having a "high ability" to read and write English (more so for women than men). When breaking this down into the original questions of being able to read and write English, we find that nearly 40% of the respondents reported that they did not read English very well or not at all, while nearly 45% did not write English very well or not at all. Of the latter, half reported "not at all." While it may be unfortunate that English literacy for Hispanic immigrants and populations may have become a political issue with many nuances and overtones, the need to reach out to Puerto Rican adults and provide them with the opportunities and help to improve English skills as an adjunct to and not a replacement of Spanish seems indicated.

The acculturation index was created by adding the weighted responses to the nine items in Table 2.3. In those cases with missing values or in instances where the question did not apply, the average obtained from all other items in the scale was substituted. The indices in items 2 through 4 described above had been recoded into quartiles; therefore, scores for the nine items ranged from 1 to 4 or 1 to 3 according to the answer options in the question.

The actual scores for the acculturation index ranged from a low of 9 to a high of 34, with the higher number indicating a greater degree of acculturation. In order to validate the acculturation scale, both internal and external validation procedures were used. An item-by-item Pearson correlation of the nine items used in the index produced correlations ranging between .18 and .75. Several external items for validation were used: born outside of mainland United States, number of years in United States, and age. Correlations of .51 ($p < .001$), .09 ($p < .01$), and -.50 ($p < .001$) were obtained for these items. In addition, the acculturation index was correlated with questions on primary ethnic self-identification and the age of the respondent when she or he came to the United States. The self-identification item asked the respondent to select among responses that ranged from "all Puerto Rican" to "all American." The correlation coefficient with this item was .43 ($p < .001$). The "age came to the US" variable was calculated using questionnaire items on year of birth and year in which the respondent came to the United States. Correlations with "age came to US" produced a coefficient of -.65 ($p < .001$). Reliability tests used to obtain Cronbach's alpha and the Guttman split-half coefficients produced an alpha of .85 and a Guttman of .80. For ease of presentation and analyses the sample was divided into groups of low, medium, and high according to their scores on the acculturation index, with approximately a third of the respondents in each group (see Table 2.4).

TABLE 2.4. Index of Acculturation by Gender

	Male		Female		Total	
	N	%	N	%	N	%
Low (score 9-16)	112	25.1	247	38.7	359	33.1
Medium (score 17-23)	164	36.8	232	36.4	396	36.5
High (score 24-34)	170	38.1	159	24.9	329	30.4
Total	446	100.0	638	100.0	1084	100.0

$\chi^2(2, N = 1084) = 29.73, p < .001.$

As noted earlier, Puerto Rican men are more integrated into the Anglo culture than are women. Males averaged a score of 20.7 and women averaged 18.9 on the acculturation index. This was significant at the .001 level ($t = 5.10$, df = 1082). How do background variables affect acculturation? There were significant correlations (ranging from .41 to .59, $p < .001$) for both males and females between acculturation and place of birth, ethnic identification, education and age in the direction expected: the longer the time in the United States, the stronger the identification as American, the higher the level of education, and the younger the respondents were the more likely they were to be acculturated. Among males the correlation between time in the United States and acculturation was low (.03). This may be due to the economic circumstances in which many Puerto Rican males (and those from other immigrant groups as well) find themselves soon after coming to the mainland. They need to find employment quickly, since many have families to support and these jobs often require a modicum of English speaking, reading, and writing abilities. Their necessary associations with Anglos can have other serendipitous effects by being in situations more often than women to hear, see, and learn other aspects of the Anglo culture. On the other hand, many women may be sheltered for longer periods of time after reaching the mainland by associations within the

Hispanic communities for their daily activities of shopping, child care, and the other household-associated activities. As they are here longer, the pressures to become bilingual and be exposed to the Anglo culture becomes just as great for the females when they too are forced to enter the labor force.

The degree of acculturation alone can be misleading if it is to be used as an explanation for behavioral consequences. The extent of one's acculturation needs to be viewed as not only what new mores and customs one is embracing in the host culture but also what mores and customs that may have served as social controls in their Puerto Rican tradition were left behind. The degree of adherence to one's tradition and roots can be a powerful influence or curb on one's behavior by serving as a social conscience in the prevention of substance abuse. This will be examined in Chapter 3.

CHAPTER 3

TRADITIONAL FAMILY VALUES

What is "traditionalism" and how does it relate to
family values? What are the family values that
concern parental responsibility in raising children?
Who do the Puerto Ricans say should be the
decision maker in the family? Should women with
small children work outside the home? Should
husbands share responsibility for housework?
Should a wife always obey her husband? Should a
wife continue her formal education after marriage?
If possible, should she choose to earn more money
than her husband does? Should boys and girls be
raised with similar attitudes about helping with
housework? Who makes the major decisions for the
family and who is responsible for the decisions for
everyday activities? How religious are they? Does
fatalism play a role in their major decisions and
problems?

TRADITION AND TRADITIONALISM

No matter how the term "values" is used in discussions of family values,
the implicit and at times explicit antecedent is the notion of "traditional."
In what sense are values traditional? As we discussed in the

Introduction, social values are the *importance* that one places on specific social acts or attitudes. These values assumedly reflect societal standards. However, in a heterogeneous and evolving society the opportunities of diverse and sometimes conflicting albeit legitimate value systems are ever present. One need only look at the enormous passions aroused in different segments of the population over the issue of abortion. To a lesser extent, there are different and often conflicting assignments of value to gambling, drinking, nonmarital sex, and homosexuality, among others, within and between many subgroups. For an insightful discussion of differences in cultural value systems and their impact on alcohol use, see Pittman (1967).

To examine any set of values and judge their impact on the individual and the rest of the community, one needs to understand and examine these values in light of the different traditions in which they have evolved. When one evokes, for example, a Judeo-Christian basis or derivation of selected family values, there is the belief that one accepts and shares with most others in the community a common heritage of unchanging family values. This value base is assumed to provide us with a clear set of guidelines or rules for present-day social behavior within and by the family. But clearly there have been many divergent familial paths within this heritage, and different cultures and subgroups have viewed and interpreted Judeo-Christian family values in their own unique ways. For orthodox and fundamentalist followers within the many divisions of Judaism and Christianity, there may be many more similarities in family values than differences, since they often strive to interpret family values as close to their original Biblical sources as possible. Indeed, they may be more similar in their value systems to their fundamentalist counterparts in the other religions than to their nonfundamentalist or more liberal brethren in both Judaism and Christianity. However, for the majority of persons in Western culture who are not fundamentalist or orthodox, only vague guidelines, often mediated by local interpretations that have accumulated over the centuries, provide the bases for determining what are the "right" or "wrong" ways for women, men, and children to behave toward each other both within and without the nuclear family structure. These guidelines are usually the traditions, the "thinking-as-usual" that is reinforced by community acquiescence and sanctions that provide the blueprints for "correct" behavior (Schutz, 1944, p. 501). This "community blueprint" we may call "traditionalism."

Traditionalism has been defined as "the attitude or philosophy that the established patterns of the past are the best guides in deciding behavior in the present and the future" (Theodorson & Theodorson, 1969, p. 441). The term "traditionalism" derives from the concept of tradition, which has been defined by Shils (1981, p. 12) as "anything which is transmitted or handed down from the past to the present....The decisive criterion is that, having been created through human actions, through thought and imagination, it is handed down from one generation to the next". Another perspective on this definition is that of Winthrop (1991, p. 300), who sees tradition as "a continuity of understanding relative to some activity, way of life, or mode of expression, which guides particular acts and beliefs."

A clear image of the role of tradition in everyday life was presented in the musical *Fiddler on the Roof* based on the Sholem Aleichem short stories about the dairyman Tevye in the fictional East European town of Karislevka (Aleichem, 1956). There, as the main song "Tradition" declares, it is tradition that dictates that the father is the breadwinner, instrumental in his daily prayers, and has the final say in the home, while his wife must be a good homemaker, keep a kosher kitchen, raise the family, and manage the household to free her husband for religious study, and the children are to be obedient while learning their adult roles as Orthodox Jewish men and women and wait for the arranged wedding match that the parents will pick out for them.

Tradition includes physical or material objects (e.g., buildings, paintings, and books) as well as conceptual or abstract things (e.g., beliefs, norms, values, and human actions). In the case of the latter there is no concrete object to hand down or transmit. What is transmitted are:

> ...the patterns or images of actions which they imply or present and the beliefs requiring, recommending, regulating, permitting, or prohibiting the reenactment of those patterns. What particular actions and complexes and sequences of actions leave behind are the conditions for subsequent actions, images in memory and documents of what they were when they happened and, under certain conditions, normative precedents or prescriptions for future actions. (Shils, 1981, p. 12)

Individuals that adhere to various aspects of tradition do not necessarily need to recognize it as something from the past. On the contrary, it may be considered and accepted as much a part of the present as recent innovations. These individuals do not accept tradition just because it has been handed down to them, but because they believe in it (Shils, 1981).

Traditions, though, do not remain unchallenged. Progress and innovation are viewed as antithetical to tradition, leading some to view adherence to traditional ways as potentially damaging or stifling to a society (Shils, 1981). The process of acculturation may be seen as a threat to tradition, for as individuals move away from the ways of their own culture to adopt the ways of the host, often tradition (at least as defined by the original culture) is abandoned. For some, becoming acculturated involves the stress of balancing what may be contradictory norms and values between their old and new cultures. Furthermore, there may be the fear that they will not be able to become fully assimilated (if that is their goal) if their traditional values distinguish them as being too different from other persons in the host culture.

This is not to say that individuals cannot remain traditional as defined by the culture in which they were born should they become acculturated to a very different society. One of the difficulties with using acculturation alone (or even in a model with sociodemographic antecedents) as an explanatory variable is that even if one is highly acculturated, this may not always be accompanied by the abandonment of the identity and value systems of the group from which one comes. Many persons in various ethnic groups, e.g., Jews, Italians, Greeks, and Chinese, may be highly acculturated but still maintain intense emotional and behavioral ties with their culture of origin and its traditions (Lieberman, 1987).

A proposition raised by these observations is that the degree of acculturation may not necessarily indicate the degree to which one loses one's traditional ethnic and cultural ties and values. It is possible, as Lieberman has suggested, that it is not what the immigrants may move *toward* in the process of acculturation, but rather *which traditional values were abandoned* that permit deviant substance use patterns to develop. In a somewhat similar approach, Gilbert (1985) has suggested that Hispanic women who are moving toward the Anglo culture, by participating more in social situations where drinking is available, alter their drinking patterns *away* from the traditional restraints that guide them.

PUERTO RICAN FAMILY VALUES

The portrayal of traditional family values within the Puerto Rican society are those most clearly ascribed to Puerto Rican women. While one may project "male chauvinist" imputations to the apparent subservient role inherent in the traditional status of many women, the values and strengths of the Hispanic family life and ties clearly illustrate Durkheim's (1984) division of labor as well as any other example. Because the Puerto Rican woman looks so consistently and passionately inward to the care and well-being of her family (as have women in most cultures), family values and beliefs have evolved that emphasize and reinforce her role as nurturer and home manager. These values, often expressed as a set of unspoken beliefs, not only serve to protect and facilitate her role vis-à-vis her family and community, but also frees her husband for the breadwinner role. On the downside, these values also may create the unintended negative or destructive social behaviors of the husband, including womanizing and heavy drinking, that are oriented more to maintaining status in the eyes of other men than to his family. Christensen (1979) has argued that despite this obviously discriminatory sex role pattern for women, the cycle of child rearing, approved by women, maintains the patterns:

> Often the very Puerto Rican woman who is discriminated against in many respects of her life repeats the same cycle in her attitude toward her children. She is apt to be accepting of mischievous *macho* and sexual behavior on the part of her boys, although she may make the proper remonstrances (often with repressed giggles). In the meantime, her girls are still raised to be obedient and nonviolent, closely supervised and protected, and with a narrowly conceived sex role. (p. 61)

This type of family belief system was summarized by Maldonado-Sierra, Trent, & Marina (1960), in a study titled "Neurosis and Traditional Family Beliefs in Puerto Rico:"

> A definition of the term *traditional Latin-American family beliefs* would include the following premises as a brief summary of the most common features: the unquestioned and absolute obedience to the father; the necessary and absolute self-sacrifice of the mother to the needs of her husband and children; the assumption of the indubitable, biological, and natural superiority of the male within the culture; the expectation of superlative femininity, including home-making, maternity, mothering, etc.; the double standard of sexual morality; the segregation of the sexes; and the like... (p. 237)

From a functional perspective, the family of the *barrio* is very much like the family of the Eastern European Jewish *shtetl*. Rather than a denigration of the female role, it is elevated as the more important role within the family—a more spiritual and martyr-like role that insists on stricter regulations and control for women than for men.

It has been suggested that these socially explicit and rigid controls over the behavior of women were instrumental in preventing Hispanic women from becoming involved in deviant behavior (Aguirre-Molina, 1991; Trotter, 1985). The ideal Hispanic woman would follow the values defined in the concept of *marianismo*, a chaste, passive and submissive woman (idealized in the Virgin Mary) who will pass on to her children, most emphatically to the daughters, the behaviors and attitudes that are expected of the individuals in that culture.

These values of *marianismo* complement the values that define the concept of *machismo* or male superiority. Adhering to a patriarchal family structure, a husband/father is expected to be the authority figure in his family, and as such he is to be respected by all of his immediate family members. He is supposed to provide financial security for his family, protect the virginity of the women in his household and family, and show his virility through the sexual conquest of women other than his wife (Ghali, 1982; Soto, 1983; Stevens, 1973).

Although some researchers have claimed that Puerto Rican women are somewhat less traditional than other Hispanic women (Aguirre-Molina, 1991; Soto, 1983), the oppressive nature of the socialization process, which does not allow women to demonstrate any aggressiveness, has been thought to cause the *mal de los nervios* or *ataques* (a malady caused by nervousness or nervous attacks) not uncommon among Puerto Rican women. A psychiatrist, Maria Oquendo (1994), described this *ataque de nervios* as "a response to acute stress found primarily in Hispanic women....Descriptions include seizure-like responses, ...dissociation, ...suicidal fits, ...and panic-like responses" (p. 60). Ghali (1982) believed that *ataques* were "a form of hysteria characterized by hyperkinetic seizures as a response to acute tension and anxiety. The *ataques* is a culturally expected reaction to situations of serious stress and can be an ordinary occurrence" (p. 99).

Ataques have been observed among Puerto Rican soldiers in stressful situation as well, marked by mutism, hyperventilation, bizarreness, hyperkinesis, uncommunicativeness, and violence (Rothenberg, 1964). The *ataque* is on some occasions socially expected and culturally reinforced as, for example, when a beloved one dies the *ataque* is seen as an indication of the depth of the sorrow (Comas-Diaz, 1987). The Puerto Rican culture therefore allows psychosomatic displays on the part of women but traditionally does not allow for their use of alcohol or drugs as self-medicating stress relievers. Oquendo (1994), observed that:

> [Puerto Rican] women are expected to accept misfortune stoically and silently. Unlike men, who may cope with such affects (anger, frustration, or fear) by direct expression or by the use of alcohol, women may be restricted to an expression that is considered uncontrollable and understandable rather than a weakness of character." (p. 60)

It has been repeatedly noted that traditional norms regarding drinking among Hispanics tend to be restrictive for women and permissive for men. These norms are not only accepted by men but by women as well. It is the group acceptance of these traditional norms that make them work and keep problem-drinking rates low among Puerto Rican women. Ullman (1958) has hypothesized the relationship of traditional norms to alcoholism by stating that,

> ...in any group or society in which the drinking customs, values and sanctions—together with the attitudes of all segments of the group or society—are well established, known to and agreed upon by all, and are consistent with the rest of the culture, the rates of alcoholism will be low. (p. 50)

Ullman's assertion does not need to be limited to the study of alcoholism but can be used as well in the study of inappropriate or problem drinking. With changes occurring regarding the independence of women economically, often due to necessity, in particular those women coming to the United States, it is clear that not only drinking attitudes but many others as well are questioned and threatened as women move to become less subservient and tolerant of the *machismo* values. As well, migration to the United States along with the progress of the women's movement have had their impacts on the traditional gender norms, more specifically on the restrictive use of alcohol, which are part of the traditional cultural norms (Comas-Diaz, 1989).

THE MEASUREMENT OF TRADITIONALISM

A review of the literature reveals that there are few studies that examine the specific items of the traditional gender roles of Hispanic women and men that are centered in the family. Among the available scales that have been created is the "traditional subscale" adopted and expanded by Maldonado-Sierra et al. (1960). This scale consists of 32 items (within a 123-item questionnaire) "aimed specifically at determining Ss' expressed acceptance of traditional Latin-American family beliefs" (Maldonado-Sierra et al., 1960). The items consist of questions regarding the role of women, men, and children in the family, as well as in relation to one another. The Attitude toward Women Scale (AWS) also has been used to measure the female sex role among Hispanics. The AWS developed by Spence and Helmreich (1972), or some variation of the scale, was found to have been used in 8 of the 10 studies conducted between 1976 and 1983 and reviewed by Vazquez-Nuttall, Romero-Garcia, & DeLeon (1987). The AWS consists "of statements describing the rights, roles and privileges women ought to have" (Vazquez-Nuttall et al., 1987, p. 413). Notwithstanding the existence and use of these scales, there is at present no standardized and generally accepted scale to measure traditional sex roles created specifically for use with both Hispanic men and women or for the subgroup of Puerto Ricans. Therefore, for purposes of this study a scale was created based on traditional sex roles as defined by the literature and drawn from the questions asked to the respondents in this study (Aguirre-Molina, 1991; Christensen, 1979; Ghali, 1982; Soto, 1983; Stevens, 1973; Trotter, 1985).

Among the information gathered were answers to questions that reflect the norms governing behavior of men and women vis-à-vis the family. Some items reflected attitudes within the full sample, while others were specific to marital role behaviors and decision-making events and were asked only of those who were married or living in a cohabitation relationship. For the full sample, respondents were asked to provide Likert-type responses (strongly agree to strongly disagree) to "should" type questions, e.g., "Husbands should make all the important decisions in a marriage." Questions for the subgroup of "married" concerned gender responsibilities in areas of child rearing, cooking, household responsibilities, and final decision-making authority that indicate traditional intrafamily values among Puerto Ricans, e.g., "In your house who usually does the washing and drying dishes?" The responses ranged from "Usually the wife or female partner" to "Usually the husband or male partner." In addition, there were items associated with traditional religious attitudes and values that were asked of all.

This delineation of at least three dimensions defining traditionalism—role attitudes, role behaviors, and role decision-making—has a degree of face validity but presents some obstacles in these analyses. While it would be important to learn how traditional role behaviors and decision making related to choices on drug and alcohol outcomes, they cannot be combined along with traditional role attitudes into a more comprehensive indicator of traditionalism, since they were asked only of married and cohabiting respondents. Comparisons of this group to the "never married" showed that they were more likely to be older, to have been born in Puerto Rico; be less educated, to have spent more time in the United States, and be less likely to have been raised in a rural environment. Nevertheless, indices of behavior and decision making are presented in addition to role attitudes, since they describe important aspects of traditionalism albeit limited to part of the population.

INDEX OF TRADITIONAL FAMILY ROLE ATTITUDES (A)

Eight questions were asked of the entire sample to elicit traditional family norms. These Likert-type questions, with response categories from "strongly agree" to "strongly disagree," were:

1. Raising children should be just as important to a man as it is to a woman.
2. Husbands should make all the important decisions in the marriage.
3. It is OK if a wife with young children has a job outside the home, if she wants.
4. Men should not do housework
5. It is OK for a wife to earn more money than her husband.
6. A wife should do whatever her husband wants.
7. Married women have a right to continue their education.
8. Only girls and not boys should help with housework.

In questions 2, 4, 6, and 8 agreement indicates the traditional belief, while in questions 1, 3, 5, and 7 disagreement represents the traditional belief. Taking into consideration the wording of the question, the values assigned to the responses "strongly agree" to "strongly disagree" were recoded so that the higher number reflected a higher level of traditional attitude. Therefore, for questions 1, 3, 5, and 7 above, "strongly agree" was assigned a value of 1 and "strongly disagree" a value of 4, while for questions 2, 4, 6, and 8 "strongly agree" was assigned a value of 4 and "strongly disagree" a value of 1.

Table 3.1 presents the frequency distributions for the items to be included in the Traditional Family Role Attitude Index. As indicated, these items reflect some of the different facets that have been used to describe traditional Hispanic families, including the Puerto Rican.

TABLE 3.1. Percent Responses for Traditional Family Role Attitudes Items
(N = 1084)

	Strongly agree	Agree	Disagree	Strongly disagree
1. Raising children should be just as important to a man as it is to a woman	68.0	29.9	1.8	0.3
2. Husbands should make all the important decisions in the marriage	7.6	20.8	53.3	16.3
3. It is OK if a wife with young children has a job outside the home, if she wants	11.8	44.0	29.1	15.1
4. Men should not do housework	2.8	12.0	62.5	22.7
5. It is OK for a wife to earn more money than her husband	25.1	59.4	13.5	2.0
6. A wife should do whatever her husband wants	2.7	16.7	61.4	19.2
7. Married women have a right to continue their education	42.0	56.4	1.2	0.4
8. Only girls, and not boys should help with housework	3.7	11.3	63.4	21.6

Questions 1 and 3 relate to the attitudes regarding responsibility for child rearing. Questions 2 and 6 concern the role of wives as submissive with respect to the husband or male partner in the house. Questions 4 and 8 relate to the tasks that females rather than males are expected to perform in the household. Questions 5 and 7 address issues of independence and power to which traditional women would not have much access.

The Traditional Family Role Attitude Index (Traditionalism A) was created by adding the responses to the eight items presented in Table 3.1. For cases with missing data, the mean of the available items for each case was substituted. A maximum possible score of 32 indicated the highest level of traditional attitudes and a score of 8 would indicate the lowest level of traditional attitudes. The actual scores ranged between 8 and 24. Pearson correlations between the variables used in the index and the Traditionalism A (Attitude) Index ranged between .31 and .61 (all relationships significant, $p < .001$). The internal reliability of the index was tested by using Cronbach's alpha and Guttman split-half coefficients. The alpha was .61 and the Guttman coefficient was .64. Traditionalism A was externally validated by using Pearson correlations with the variables of Age and Place of Birth (where born in Puerto Rico was assigned a value of 1 and born in the United States or other country was assigned a value of 2 and 3, respectively). The coefficient with Age was .24, and the coefficient with Place of Birth was -.20 (both statistically significant, $p < .001$). In addition, the index was validated with ethnic self-identification (the largest weight score was assigned to "all American" and the lowest "all Puerto Rican") and time in the United States. Traditionalism A correlated negatively with ethnic identity ($r = -.07, p < .05$), however, Traditionalism A was not related to "time in the US" ($r = .02, p > .05$).

TABLE 3.2. Index of Traditional Family Role Attitudes (Traditionalism A) by Gender

	Male		Female		Total	
	N	%	N	%	N	%
Low traditional (score 8–14)	110	24.7	252	39.5	362	33.4
Medium traditional (score 15–16)	135	30.3	185	29.0	320	29.5
High traditional (score 17–24)	201	45.0	201	31.5	402	37.1
Total	446	100.0	638	100.0	1084	100.0

$\chi^2(2, N = 1084) = 30.46, p < .001$.

TABLE 3.3. Acculturation and Traditionalism A Score Means by Gender
(N = 1084)

	Mean	t Value	2-tail significance
Acculturation			
Male	20.7		
Female	18.9	5.10	.000
Traditionalism A			
Male	16.1		
Female	15.1	6.02	.000

For some of the analyses and for ease of presentation, the index was collapsed into groups of low, medium and high according to their Traditional Family Role Attitude Index scores with approximately a third of the respondents in each group. This is presented in Table 3.2 comparing females and males.

If we compare the results presented in Table 3.2 with the Index of acculturation in Table 2.4, we note that Puerto Rican men are not only more likely to be more traditional (score high) than Puerto Rican women, they are also more likely to be more acculturated than the women. These differences are significant at the .001 level and the t-test results are presented in Table 3.3.

Pearson correlations between the Indices of Acculturation and Traditionalism A were relatively low (-.2894) for the entire sample. They were slightly higher for the females (-.3479) than for the males (-.2922). Based on these correlations, the finding that some Puerto Rican men scored high on Traditionalism A as well as on the Index of Acculturation (as did some women) underscores what has been suggested before: that acculturation does not necessarily mean the loss of traditional values for all persons. One also might speculate that because traditional values allow for more freedom for Puerto Rican men than for Puerto Rican women, men are less conflicted by the results of acculturation. These relationships between acculturation and traditionalism will be further explored in Chapter 7.

FAMILY DECISION MAKING AND MARITAL ROLE RESPONSIBILITIES

Eighteen questions were asked only of those respondents who were married or in a cohabitation relationship (410 persons, 37.9%). This was to determine who in the family had the responsibility for household tasks and who was the final authority when it came to decision-making situations related to everyday activities. These items represent the most common elements of the Puerto Rican marital role norms for household responsibilities. For each situation, the respondents were given a choice of answers: "usually the wife (or female partner)," "usually the husband (or male partner)," "both together," "either one or the other but not together," or "neither the husband nor the wife." The 18 questions and responses to these items are presented in Table 3.4.

These items reflect some of the different traditional marital role assignments for behaviors found in most families in Western culture, including Hispanics. Items 9 through 13 are female responsibilities in traditional Puerto Rican households, while items 1 through 7 and 15 through 18 were traditionally assigned to the male.

Questions 8 and 14 are more difficult to clearly assign to the male or female roles for different reasons. While grocery shopping is usually seen in the traditional family as a function of the housewife's skill and knowledge in kitchen matters, she is often accompanied or constricted by her husband or male partner who is the keeper of the purse and who has the ultimate say in the matter. Thus, for purposes of categorizing in the construction of the index, we will consider this a male responsibility. Disciplining the children may call for either the mother or the father taking the lead for dispensing the consequences (the father more likely to respond to the more severe infractions). However, for everyday disciplining, it was more likely that the wife (or female

TABLE 3.4. Percent Responses for Traditional Family Decision Making and
Role Responsibility Items (for Married and Cohabiting)

	Wife	Husband	Both	Either	N
Who usually makes the final decision about...					
1. what house or apartment to take	14.9	21.0	63.4	0.7	409
2. how much life insurance and what type	8.4	24.4	66.1	1.1	356
3. whether the wife (female partner) should be employed at all	27.6	14.8	56.2	1.4	352
4. whether the husband (male partner) changes his job or not	3.0	50.7	44.4	1.9	363
5. where to spend vacations; where to go on outings	6.0	11.1	80.9	2.0	398
6. what improvements should be made around the house	30.8	11.7	57.0	0.5	402
7. which school the children should go to	18.4	7.0	66.5	8.1	272
In your house, who usually...					
8. does the grocery shopping	39.2	14.0	45.5	1.3	393
9. does the cooking	80.7	3.8	7.5	8.0	398
10. washes clothes	88.7	3.3	6.2	1.8	400
11. washes and dries dishes	72.2	4.1	14.0	9.7	392
12. bathes children	83.5	1.5	7.0	8.0	199
13. fixes breakfast	73.5	8.3	7.1	11.1	396
14. disciplines children	18.4	7.0	66.5	8.1	272
15. cleans the car	3.6	82.4	10.8	3.2	222
16. takes car to be repaired or repairs car	0.9	92.5	3.8	2.8	212
17. attends to furniture repair	11.3	72.3	14.8	1.6	311
18. purchases expensive items (i.e. car, TV, furniture, etc.)	6.2	33.9	58.1	1.8	387

partner) would have been responsible. Thus, we will consider item 14 a
female responsibility.

When we examine the responses of the mainland Puerto Ricans, we
find that those items that were traditionally assigned to the male in

Puerto Rico were actually more likely to carried out jointly (except for items 4 and 18, although women have a great deal of input). We believe that this reflects a perceived Anglo normative role for women in having a greater voice in the family and appearing more egalitarian. When it comes to the traditionally female in-home tasks, however, women still carry the burden except for the ambiguous issue of disciplining children. While there is no clear explanation for the discipline issue, it is possible that the streets of New York City and the more rapid acculturation of youth results in more serious actions by children than was true in the more traditional communities of Puerto Rico.

In order to create the index, a value of 3 (indicating the more traditional direction) was assigned to each response of "husband" for the male-assigned items, as was "wife" for the female items. If a male assigned item was carried out by the female or a female assigned item carried out by a male, a score of 1 (indicating less traditional) was given. (In all items, if the respondents chose "both together" or "either one but not together" an intermediate score of two was assigned.)

Factor analysis with varimax rotation of the 18 items was used to determine which variables were to be kept for the index. This resulted in two distinct factors. Factor one (family decision making) explained 18.3% of the variance with an eigenvalue of 3.30. Factor loadings ranged from .51758 to .73703. Factor two (role behavior) explained 13.5% of the variance with an eigenvalue of 2.43. Factor loadings ranged from .44445 to .76408. As a consequence of the factor analysis, two indices were created: decision making and role behavior.

INDEX OF TRADITIONAL FAMILY DECISION MAKING (D)

The Traditional Family Decision Making Index was created by adding the scores of each of the seven items in factor one (1, 2, 3, 5, 6, 7, and, 18). A maximum possible score of 21 would indicate the highest level of traditional male decision-making responsibility and a score of 7 would indicate the lowest level of traditional decision making regarding family situations. Pearson correlations between the variables used in the index and the Traditionalism D (Family Decision Making) index ranged between .56 and .74 (all relationships significant, $p < .001$). The internal reliability of the index was tested by using Cronbach's alpha (.76) and the Guttman split-half coefficient (.68). To validate the index externally two variables were used: Age of the respondent and Place of birth (Puerto Rico = 1, US or other = 2). Age was not found to correlate with traditional family decision making ($r = .05, p > .05$); nevertheless Place of Birth was ($r = -18, p < .001$). This suggests that an individuals' age is not as important regarding adherence to traditional family decision making as was having been born on "the Island" where the traditional norms would have been enforced more consistently and therefore would have been internalized more strongly than for those born in the United States or elsewhere.

For some of the analyses the index will be collapsed into groups of low, medium, and high according to their index scores with approximately a third of the respondents in each group (see Table 3.5).

TABLE 3.5.   Index of Traditional Family Decision-Making (D) by Gender

| | Male | | Female | | Total | |
Frequency	N	%	N	%	N	%
Low traditional (score 7–13)	74	29.2	54	38.0	128	32.4
Medium traditional (score 14)	81	32.0	41	28.9	122	30.9
High traditional (score 15–21)	98	38.8	47	33.1	145	36.7
Total	253	100.0	142	100.0	395	100.0

$\chi^2(2, N = 395) = 3.24, p > .05.$

INDEX OF TRADITIONAL FAMILY ROLE BEHAVIOR (B)

The Traditional Family Role Behavior Index was created by adding the responses of each of the five items discerned as factor two (items 9, 11, 10, 13, and 8). A maximum possible score of 15 would indicate the highest level of traditional family role behavior and a score of 5 would indicate the lowest level of traditional behavior regarding household task assignments. Pearson correlations between the variables used in the index and the Traditionalism B (Behavior) Index ranged between .59 and .74 (all relationships significant, $p < .001$). The internal reliability of the Index was tested by using Cronbach's alpha (.71) and the Guttman split-half coefficient (.70). The Traditional Family Role Behavior Index was externally validated by Pearson correlation with time in the United States ($r = -.18$, $p < .001$). Age, as was the case with traditional family decision making, and place of birth did not significantly correlate with traditional role behavior. This supports the finding that age alone cannot be used as a presumptive factor on level of adherence to traditional norms of the culture.

For some of the analyses the Traditional Sex Role Behavior Index will be dichotomized rather than trichotomized because of the skewing of scores at the high end (see Table 3.6).

Table 3.6. Index of Traditional Family Role Behavior (B) by Gender

Frequency	Males		Females		Totals	
	N	%	N	%	N	%
Low traditional (score 5–13)	126	47.9	55	37.9	181	44.4
High traditional (score 14,15)	137	52.1	90	62.1	227	55.6
Total	263	100.0	145	100.0	408	100.0

$\chi^2(1, N = 408) = 3.99, p > .05.$

SPIRITUAL INFLUENCES

Two additional cultural themes that are deeply rooted in the Hispanic traditions are religiosity and fatalism. The impact of fatalism and religiosity on psychosocial disorders and other health-related issues including treatment has been noted by several researchers (Byrd, Cohn, Gonzalez, Parada, & Cortes, 1999; Cuadrado, 1998; Harmon, Castro, & Coe, 1996; Neff & Hoppe, 1993; Vazquez-Nuttall et al., 1984). Neff and Hoppe (1993) view fatalism and religiosity as complementary resources, reflecting the individual's perception of little control over life (fatalism) as a personal resource when coupled with high religiosity, thus promoting social strength through the integration of the two:

> Thus, though fatalism may imply a lack of perceived individual control, typically associated with depression, negative effects of fatalism may be offset by religious involvement. In contrast, the fatalistic individual, less integrated into religious activities (i.e., lacking both personal and social resources) may be the most distressed. For less fatalistic (i.e., high mastery) individuals, religiosity may provide an additional source of support or protection. The less fatalistic individual who is less integrated into religious activities may lack the social buffer but may possess personal resources. (p. 6)

They go on to point out that this is particularly true for low acculturated persons (Neff & Hoppe, 1993, p. 18). Castro and Gutierres (1997) also have argued for the value of including fatalism and religiosity, in combination, along with other cultural variables specifically for the study of such outcomes as substance abuse:

> Acculturation has been regarded as an important moderating and mediating variable that is associated with health outcomes among Mexican-Americans and other Hispanics. For example, one study argues that Mexican culture increases depression because it promotes an external locus of control orientation (fatalism). On the other hand, these fatalistic external attributions may protect self-esteem and reduce anxiety by releasing the person from social demands for achievement and success. In

addition, responsibility to the group rather than to one's self may promote depression but relieve anxiety because of the reciprocal social support provided by the family or social group. Even though this study suggests provocative associations between Mexican culture and psychological well-being, it raises questions about the social dynamics that influence the well-being of Mexican-Americans and how these factors might promote drug use and abuse. (pp. 512–513)

To learn more about the influence of religiosity and fatalism upon substance abuse outcomes among Puerto Ricans, indices reflecting these components were also created.

RELIGIOSITY

A large majority of the sample was Catholic (80.5%), but significant differences were found between men and women. Males were more likely to say that they were other than Catholic (23.5% of men and 16.7% of women, $p < .01$, including "no affiliation") and were almost twice as likely as women to cite no affiliation (9.1% vs. 5.1%).

An important element of traditionalism results from the influence that religion has on one's values and lifestyle, since religion is often the perceived underpinning of correct and appropriate behaviors. Nearly three quarters of the sample said that religion is "very important" in their lives, more so for women (77.3%) than men (63.7% $p < .001$).

We also found that 83.8% of the persons who stated that religion is a very important part of their lives now came from homes where religion also was important, with no significant differences between men and women. Although 90.9% of the sample attributed at least some importance to religion in their lives, only 45.6% attended religious services once a month or more often. Women were more likely to report attending religious services at least once a month than men were (51.2% vs. 37.5%, $p < .001$). A large majority of the sample (72.7%) stated that they prayed every day, but there was a considerable difference between the males and females (59.4% vs. 81.9%, $p < .001$). Most respondents

(91.8%) believed that religious training is as important as education but there was a significant difference between men and women (85.7% vs. 96.1%, $p < .001$).

The Index of Religiosity was created by adding the scores assigned to responses for the religiosity questions:

1. How important is religion in your life?
   Very important (score 1)
   Somewhat important (score 2)
   Not really important (score 3)
   Not at all important (score 4)

2. About how often do you attend religious services?
   Once a week or more (score 1)
   1 – 2 times a month (score 2)
   A few times a year (score 3)
   Rarely (score 4)
   Never (score 5)

3. How often do you pray?
   Every day (score 1)
   Once a week (score 2)
   A few times a month (score 3)
   A few times a year (score 4)
   Never (score 5)

4. I think religious training is just as important as formal education for children.
   Agree (score 1)
   Disagree (score 4)

The resulting score ranged from 4 (indicating highest level of religiosity) to 18 (lowest level of religiosity). The index was validated by Cronbach's alpha of .69 and a Guttman split-half of .62. For purposes of analysis and

TABLE 3.7. Index of Religiosity by Gender

	Male		Female		Total	
Score	N	%	N	%	N	%
Low (score 8 – 18)	213	48.0	148	23.5	361	33.6
Medium (score 6,7)	92	20.7	196	31.1	288	26.8
High (score 4,5)	139	31.3	286	45.4	425	39.6
Total	444	100.0	630	100.0	1074	100.0

$\chi^2(2, N = 1074) = 69.99, p < .001.$

presentation, the variable was trichotomized. In the recode process, the direction of the scores also was adjusted so that a higher number of 3 was assigned to "high" religiosity (see Table 3.7). In Table 3.7, we find that women are considerably more likely than men to indicate that they are religious (45.4% vs. 31.0%). At the low end of the scale, the differences are even more pronounced (48.0% of the males vs. 23.5% of the females).

FATALISM

All respondents were asked five questions that tapped whether or not they had a sense of control over their destiny:

1. Do you think it's better to plan your life a good ways ahead, or would you say life is too much a matter of luck to plan ahead very far?

2. When you do make plans ahead, do you usually get to carry out things the way you expected, or do things usually come up to change your plans?

3. Have you usually felt pretty sure your life would work out the way you want it to, or have there been times when you haven't been sure about it?

4. Some people feel they can run their lives pretty much the way they want to; others feel the problems of life are sometimes too big for them. Which one are you most like?

5. When you have a problem, do you make a plan of action and follow it, or try to take your mind off your problem for a while?

These items were correlated with each other and ranged from .14 to .44, all significant at $p < .001$. It is said to be "common wisdom" in the Puerto Rican community that women are more fatalistic (as well as religious) than men. This was found to be true for each of the above items.

All questions were asked with only the two-response categories presented. Answers were scored 1 or 2 with the second possible response being assigned a higher score indicating greater fatalism. Scores were added to create an index of fatalism. The index was validated by a Cronbach's alpha of .64 and a Guttman split-half coefficient of .60. Mean comparison between males and females showed that females were significantly more fatalistic than males ($M = 2.02$ vs. $M = 1.65$, respectively, $t = -4.00$, df = 1082, $p < .001$). The index was grouped into high, medium, and low fatalism, consisting of approximately a third of the sample in each group. The grouped Index of Fatalism is presented in Table 3.8.

TABLE 3.8. Index of Fatalism by Gender

	Male		Female		Total	
Score	N	%	N	%	N	%
Low (score 0)	132	29.6	130	20.4	262	23.6
Medium (score 1,2)	181	40.6	258	40.4	439	39.7
High (score 3–5)	133	29.8	250	39.2	383	36.7
Total	446	100.0	638	100.0	1084	100.0

$\chi^2(2, N = 1074) = 15.75, p < .001$.

How does fatalism relate to religiosity? It appears that religiosity has a negative correlation with fatalism. In Table 3.9, we see that persons who scored high on the Index of Religiosity were more likely to score low on fatalism.

This inverse relationship is true for both men and women, but more so for women ($N = 444$, $r = -.10$, $p < .05$ for men; $N = 630$, $r = -.17$, $p < .001$ for women). This finding is similar to one reported among an older black sample (Krause & Van Tran, 1989). This negative relationship is an important consideration for treatment providers when working with a Hispanic population, since as stated above by Neff and Hoppe (1993), the "negative effects of fatalism may be offset by religious involvement." Put another way, strong religious beliefs may increase one's perception of the control over their own lives despite their fatalistic outlook by instilling ideas of the course of action to be taken in one's life, the rewards that will be achieved by doing so, and the help that may follow from institutional and traditional prayer.

TABLE 3.9. Fatalism by Religiosity for Males and Females[a]

	Religiosity							
	Male				Female			
	Low	Med	High	Total	Low	Med	High	Total
Fatalism	%	%	%	%	%	%	%	%
Low	25.4	28.3	37.4	29.7	10.8	15.8	26.3	20.3
Medium	40.4	39.1	41.0	40.3	39.9	41.3	39.5	40.2
High	34.3	32.6	21.6	30.0	49.3	42.9	32.2	39.5
	$N = 444, r = -.10, p < .05$				$N = 630, r = -.17, p < .001$			

[a]Religiosity and fatalism are grouped into discrete categories for the purpose of presentation. Correlations were obtained from unrecoded versions of the variables.

CHAPTER 4

SUBSTANCE USE OUTCOMES

What are the main explanations for alcohol and drug abuse among Hispanics? How do we operationalize and measure alcohol extent and patterns of use, drinking problems, and drug use? How do background factors relate to substance use outcomes?

ALCOHOL AS BEVERAGE AND PROBLEM

Alcohol has been an important part of human history since ancient times. It has been found to play a role in early human social development (Chafetz & Demone, 1962). The functions of alcohol have been described as religious, ceremonial, hedonistic, and utilitarian (Pittman, 1967). Its religious functions can be found throughout the Bible and other literature, as well as part of sacraments in Judaism and Christianity; its ceremonial functions can be viewed through the use of beverage alcohol in events ranging from the celebration of birth to the grieving of death; its hedonistic function is found in the pleasurable feeling that the individual can experience from mealtime and recreational drinking; and the utilitarian functions are found in the stress relief and medicinal benefits that individuals in some cultures obtain from it. The function of alcohol has been described in general terms by de Ortiz (1981) as,

> ...associated with and valued for its function as behavior modifier, and for diminishing social distance and strengthening group bonds. In the former, mild consumption promotes the expression of individually and socially shared values such as relief and relaxation from fatigue, tension, apathy, and a sense of isolation. In the latter, it is expressed through ritual functions symbolizing status changes such as births, marriages, new jobs, coming of age and bereavement. (p. 3)

Thus, alcohol provides societies with important benefits. However, inappropriate or excessive use (as defined differently by the separate cultures) may cause effects that are considered opposite to the functions attributed to alcohol. That is, inappropriate or excessive use may modify behavior in ways that are not accepted by others in the society, and in that way increase social distance and isolation. In order to study problem drinking then, there must be an understanding of acceptable drinking practices within the culture of the individual or group being studied. However, we must emphasize that the purpose of this study is not to focus on alcohol abuse among Puerto Ricans, but rather, to study drinking practices—only some of which may be deemed as problematic within the framework of the traditional Puerto Rican culture—and their relationships to acculturation and traditional values.

In his discussion of the attitudes a culture may have regarding drinking Pittman (1967) defined four cultural positions: abstinent, ambivalent, permissive, and overpermissive. The abstinent culture "...is negative and prohibitive toward any type of ingestion of alcoholic beverages." The ambivalent culture has attitudes toward alcohol that conflict with other values in the culture or the attitudes of two legitimate social groups are conflicting. The permissive culture is permissive "... toward ingesting alcohol... but negative toward drunkenness and other drinking pathologies." The overpermissive culture "is permissive toward drinking, to behavior which occurs when intoxicated, and to drinking pathologies." The latter type, Pittman notes, "does not occur completely in societies, but only approximations..." where drunkenness is accepted only under certain circumstances such as special celebrations (Pittman, 1967 p. 5).

Pittman's culture classifications of the different types of attitudes toward drinking appear to be more relevant to the drinking of men than to the drinking of women even today. Even among permissive and overpermissive cultures, women's drinking tends to be regulated more stringently than men's drinking. In the traditional Puerto Rican culture the attitudes toward female drinking may be better classified outside of the Pittman schema as "restrictive–permissive." That is, although the drinking among traditional Puerto Rican women is rigidly controlled by the culture, it is not totally forbidden if it occurs within a specific context, such as the baptism of a child or a wedding. However, not all gatherings of family and/or friends are considered acceptable occasions for women to drink. More often in traditional households, alcoholic beverages will be offered only to male guests, while female guests will be offered coffee or soft drinks. The traditional woman is not expected to offer other women alcoholic beverages just as she will not expect others to offer them to her. These and similar behavioral norms have been proffered as an explanation for the low rates of drinking found among Puerto Rican women when compared to male drinking (Aguirre-Molina, 1991). Some of these norms will be presented and analyzed in the discussion of drinking in different settings presented later in this chapter.

EXPLANATIONS AND THEORIES OF HISPANIC ALCOHOL ABUSE

Studies of Hispanic alcohol and drug use generally tend to indicate that the problems of substance use and negative consequences are high among the Hispanic population and in many instances higher than other ethnic minorities and the Anglo population. However, many of these studies suffer from not being representative of the collectivity of the many Hispanic groups in the United States. For example, most researchers in this area have sampled mainly low-income or *barrio* populations, or specialized homogeneous groups, such as gangs, criminals, drug addicts or alcoholics in treatment, and so on, rather than drawing from the general populations.

Even in large national surveys, the number of respondents from Hispanic groups other than Mexican, e.g., Cuban and Puerto Rican, may be too small for statistically significant comparisons to account for variations in patterns and problems across different groups (Caetano, 1985, p. 161). In general, results tend to indicate that Hispanic men have more problems in substance use and abuse than women, but that women may be catching up (Estrada, 1982; Perez et al., 1980; Rachal et al., 1975; Sanchez-Dirks, 1978; Wilsnack & Wilsnack, 1978). Some Hispanic groups may have more of a problem than others, but because of conflicting findings, conclusions in this area are not reliable. In sum, although much suggestive and insightful research on Hispanics exists, the in-depth studies of separate groups using representative random samples remain for future researchers.

What may account for Hispanic problematic drinking? Explanations found in the literature tend to specify a number of social and psychological factors as antecedent or explanatory variables to account for these problems: education, poverty, the breakdown of proscriptive norms for women, tolerance of male drinking and drunkenness, self-medication, lack of social integration (anomie) and a loss of institutional control, and acculturation alone as explanation.

EDUCATION

Many researchers have considered these factors separately with an understanding that they are usually interconnected through the process of acculturation itself. Increased education, for example, has been correlated with increased prevalence of alcohol use among Hispanic women but not for men (Caetano, 1984b; Canino, Burnam, & Caetano, 1992; Fernandez-Pol, Bluestone, Morales, & Mizruchi, 1985; Gilbert & Cervantes, 1986). Could this association be a product of changes in the norms associated with the role of women, itself a function of acculturation, or due to exposure to Anglo drinking opportunities, also a function of acculturation, as is education? The dynamics of the interrelationships between these variables as with many others under study are complex and require careful analyses before drawing conclusions.

POVERTY

Findings from studies focusing on socioeconomic levels appear to contradict one another and highlight the problems of analysis and correlations of variables. In a study of nearly 1000 Mexican-American high school youth in the lower Rio Grande Valley region of Texas, Guinn (1978) found that "There was no evidence of any consistent relationship between socioeconomic level and alcohol use. No significant trends could be established between parent's educational or occupational levels and reported use" (p. 90). On the other hand, Alcocer (1977) reported that poverty was related to alcohol problems. It is possible that analyses of correlations at different stages of the respondent's acculturation process could result in apparently opposite conclusions (Alcocer, 1977), or that inclusion of other variables in models would also be useful.

In his study of Anglos, Spanish Americans, and American Indians Graves (1967) found that:

Relatively high rates of drinking and deviant behavior occur among Spanish–Americans *only* for relatively acculturated subjects with *low* economic access to the new goals they have adopted. Non–acculturated Spanish–Americans tend to have relatively low drinking and deviance rates *regardless* of their degree of economic access. (p. 312)

In other words, the stress of not being able to obtain desired goals in the new culture (Merton, 1968) was a factor only for those individuals who had become acculturated. Graves (1967) also hypothesized that: "...rates of observed heavy drinking and associated social problems will co–vary *negatively* with the strength of the social and psychological control structures into which respondents are mapped" (p. 315) and suggests that marriage, church, formal and informal groups are these structures. He concludes, among other things, that "...if the controls against deviance are traditionally strong, problem behavior may not be in evidence despite an increase in pressure for its display" (Graves, 1967, p. 316). Thus, it may be the loss of *traditional values as controls* rather than the stress due to acculturation that is most instrumental.

THE BREAKDOWN OF PROSCRIPTIVE NORMS FOR WOMEN

Cultural control over Hispanic female drinking is a frequent citation in the literature, but this explanation has two important issues embedded within. In one study, older Cuban Americans reported having strong negative feelings about women who drank heavily because it "...violated the ideal of the Cuban woman as the demure and voiceless mainstay of the household" (Page, Rio, Sweeney, & McKay, 1985, p. 320) and appears to be the main reason for the lack of regular female drinkers among the respondents of that study. However, another study emphasizes not the internalized norm as social control but possible fear of community response to excessive drinking: "The extremely high rate of abstinence in barrio women undoubtedly reflects strong negative sanctions against drinking....Women who drink, particularly heavy drinkers, face strong negative sanctions from family, friends and community" (Maril & Zavaleta, 1979, p. 483). The main issue—internalized control or fear of being caught—is a longtime issue for scholars trying to explain many types of deviant behavior. At times the controls (at least for women) seem rooted in extreme stereotypes of the consequences of female drinking:

> According to traditional standards of drinking behavior, Cuban men had a somewhat greater latitude than women, being allowed to patronize taverns (the only women who would do such a thing were prostitutes) and to come home drunk on isolated occasions (a drunk woman was almost certain to have compromised herself sexually). (Page et al., 1985, p. 320)

These strong views are also held within the traditional Puerto Rican community.

TOLERANCE OF MALE DRINKING AND DRUNKENNESS

Research literature indicating any existence of socially derived internalized controls restricting Hispanic male drinkers is scarce but shows up for at least one Hispanic community. Cuban men traditionally had social controls inhibiting drunkenness related to a socially derived need for control over one's physical and mental capacities, thereby setting limits for drinking (Page et al., 1985). Although some Cuban writers criticized the drinking values of the Cuban lower classes and portrayed their drinking in terms of depravity, research in Miami indicates that the lower classes may have had the same restraints as middle and upper classes (Hoffman, 1994; Page et al., 1985; Panitz et al., 1983; Stevens, 1973).

A common explanation for male excessive drinking and one frequently heard among counselors working with Hispanic problem drinkers is that *machismo* dictates that males should have the ability to consume much alcohol (Sandoval & De la Roza, 1986). Thus, cultural brakes on excessive drinking is not likely to exist and that fact (coupled with a deteriorating self image due to the weakening of the central authority role of the father in mainland United States) will result in depression and anxiety with attempts at self-medication (Panitz et al., 1983). However, Johnson and Matre (1978) point out that traditional views of *machismo* in Hispanic cultures did not include the norm that a man necessarily *had* to drink excessively. On the contrary, *indecente or* "undignified" drunkenness also violated male norms (Johnson & Matre, 1978). This will be elaborated upon in Chapter 8.

SELF-MEDICATION

The use of alcohol (and other substances as well) for the relief of the stresses due to the acculturation process also has been cited as one of the elements in the etiology of alcohol abuse in Hispanic populations (Gilbert, 1985; Gilbert & Cervantes, 1986; Laureano & Poliandro, 1991). However, for at least one group, this theory is challenged:

> ...Elderly Cuban women are often under the general stress of forced immigration combined with the specifically alcohol-related condition of living in poverty...and lack recourse to relatives or friends to cope with their predicament. If drinking were an acceptable strategy for mediating stress among Cuban women, we might expect to see some older Cuban women consuming alcohol regularly. In fact, we do not, because of their cultural background of Cuban drinking values." (Page et al., 1985, p. 327)

The observations of these researchers seem to suggest that abusive drinking among at least some immigrant Hispanics and their children is less related to stress due to acculturation than to cultural adaptation without the traditional limit setting values that had been present for traditional Hispanic women. A question raised by this is related to the main focus of this volume. Is the inappropriate, excessive, or problematic drinking of Hispanic women more closely related to acculturation and its consequences or the weakening of adherence to traditional norms, irrespective of the degree of acculturation?

LACK OF SOCIAL INTEGRATION (ANOMIE) AND LOSS OF INSTITUTIONAL CONTROL

In 1967, Graves had hypothesized that "when pressures for engaging in deviant behavior are controlled, rates of observed heavy drinking and associated social problems will co-vary *negatively* with the strength of the social and psychological control structures into which respondents are mapped" (p. 315) and [following the seminal thinking of Durkheim (1951)] suggested that marriage, church, formal and informal groups are these structures. Graves concluded, among other things, "...if controls against deviance are traditionally strong, problem behavior may not be in evidence despite an increase in pressure for its display" (Graves, 1967, p. 318). These institutions with their traditional norms will appear quite different once the immigrant comes to mainland United States, and through the process of acculturation has to adapt to a somewhat different set of norms. However, if the hold of traditional values weakens, will the barrio women maintain their high rate of abstinence? Again, this raises questions about simple acculturation models as explanations unless they also take into consideration the maintenance or loss of traditional values.

ACCULTURATION ALONE AS EXPLANATION

Acculturation, as a measure of integration into the Anglo culture, has been found to be positively related to more intensive drinking patterns for both men and women, but especially for women (Caetano, 1984a,b, 1987a,b; Marin & Posner, 1995). In comparing the drinking patterns and problems of a Mexican-American sample with one from the state of Michoacan, Mexico, to assess the impact of acculturation, Caetano and his researchers concluded, "...the general effect of acculturation among women, contrary to what happens among men, is to increase drinking problems" (Caetano & Medina Mora, 1988, p 469).

Explanations of Mexican-American alcohol misuse and abuse based on elements of the acculturation process are tempting but unclear as to their being the paramount factors. For example, there is the intriguing suggestion that much of Mexican-American alcohol abuse stems from the desire of these men and women to take on the Anglo culture without acceptance by the Anglos, but yet recognizing their being rejected by their own ethnic group because of the movement toward acculturation (Madsen, 1964). This raises the question of whether this resulting stress is due more to the failure of acceptance by the Anglos or to the insecurities of the breakdown of traditional values uniting Mexican Americans to their past or some combination of the two.

Whether any of these simpler models of explanation is sufficient to explain the substance abuse outcomes for Puerto Ricans is doubtful. As Caetano has succinctly observed:

> Unfortunately, simple models relying on only one factor (e.g., machismo) to explain drinking patterns cannot account for the variations observed in drinking behaviors among Hispanics. To understand the complexity of alcohol use among members of that ethnic group, a multifactorial model is needed that takes into account social, economic, cultural, and historical aspects of Hispanic life in the United States. (Caetano, Clark, & Tam, 1998, p. 235)

It also has been noted that even in the absence of acculturation, change may occur among members of the more traditional society that parallel the effects of acculturation: In a study of three-generationally linked Mexican-American families in San Antonio, Texas, the authors conclude that in the younger generation women, language acculturation is linked with more intensive drinking patterns, but they also note that alcohol consumption among younger women in Mexico also has increased despite the absence of acculturation issues (Markides et al., 1988). What is absent from the literature is any clear study of the effect of the loss of traditional values within the culture of origin itself.

EXPLANATIONS AND THEORIES OF HISPANIC DRUG ABUSE

Explanations for Hispanic drug use have focused more on situational factors than on levels of acculturation or loss of traditional norms. Booth, Castro, & Anglin (1990) outline factors that have been found to be particularly relevant to the Hispanic drug use experience: a disruptive family environment, drug availability, peer influence, and unconventional behavior (e.g., rebelliousness, prostitution and early sexual activity). *Machismo* itself has been targeted as an explanation in a somewhat different manner than for alcohol use. In a study of male Mexican heroin addicts along the Mexican border just south of Arizona, Quintero and Estrada (1998) suggest that

> The aggressive aspects of machismo provide the *tecato* [male heroin addicts] with an effective means of adapting to a social lifeworld fraught with personal risks. Through enacting & recreating the ideal of machismo in his day-to-day interactions, the *tecato* gains social status as well as a means of self-defense and a strategy for drug use management. (p. 3)

These factors, although found to be strongly related to drug use, do not necessarily explain drug use, and it is reasonable to suggest that they represent symptoms of the complex problems emerging from acculturation and the loss of traditional controls and inhibitors of illicit drug use.

Research on drug use among Puerto Ricans in the general population, as is true of the other Hispanic groups, has been limited. Available research usually reflects institutionalized populations such as addicts in treatment or prison or predisposition toward drug use in adolescent populations. Explanations for drug use among different Hispanic groups have followed mainly the logic of acculturation alone or stress factors related to acculturation (Amaro et al., 1990; Szalay et al., 1993; Velez & Ungemack, 1989). Another possible explanation (although not systematically studied) is based on the loss of traditional norms. This is an outgrowth of the observation that for women, the traditional

Hispanic culture has restrictive and near-prohibitive norms regarding alcohol (Aguirre-Molina, 1991). However, with regard to drug use, there are no specific traditional norms for either men or women to abandon. What then can be rejected within the traditional norm structure that *may* be conducive to drug abuse? Our answer, throughout this volume, is that it is not necessarily the adherence to or lack of *specific* regulatory norms that may affect drug and alcohol use behaviors in mainland United States but rather adherence or rejection of a more general traditional outlook particularly as it relates to the definition of gender role behavior of Puerto Rican men and women. The data to support this will be presented in Chapters 6 and 7.

Several studies have suggested that within the acculturation process experienced by Puerto Rican men and women stress is produced due to cultural differences, the language barrier, and ethnic discrimination to which the individual may be exposed, and that stress may be relieved through the use of drugs (Berry, 1980; Gilbert, 1985; Linsky, Colby, & Straus, 1986). In their comparison of drug use among Puerto Rican juveniles with different degrees of exposure to New York City culture, Velez & Ungemack (1989) found that as the degree of exposure to the culture increased so did the likelihood of using drugs.

Language knowledge and preference are among the first factors examined to determine an individual's level of acculturation. In their study of 339 Mexican youths in East Los Angeles, Perez et al. (1980) found that language used at home and/or with peers was related to use of drugs:

> ...language use in the home presents a consistent relationship with drug use. As one moves into groups of more frequent users of drugs, one uniformly observes more English spoken. PCP is commonly considered a more serious and dangerous drug than either marijuana or alcohol. It is of interest to note that users of PCP report more use of English than users of either marijuana or alcohol. (p. 632)

Amaro et al. (1990) drew upon data from the 1982–1984 Hispanic

Health and Nutrition Evaluation Survey to study this relationship
between acculturation and illicit drug use among Hispanics:

> In both Mexican Americans and Puerto Ricans, language use was
> significantly associated with marijuana use in the previous year....The
> odds of using marijuana were eight times greater for Mexican Americans
> and five times greater for Puerto Ricans who were English–speaking than
> among Spanish–speakers....The odds of using cocaine were 25 times
> greater among Mexican Americans who scored toward the
> English–dominant end of the language use index than among those who
> were Spanish–dominant. Among Puerto Ricans, English–speakers were
> two times more likely than were Spanish–speakers to report cocaine use in
> the previous year, but the association was weak. (p. 57)

In their study of the impact of gender and acculturation on illicit
drug use among individuals of Mexican origin in Fresno, California,
Vega et al. (1998) also measured acculturation by assessing English
versus Spanish language preference. They found that higher levels of
acculturation and being born in the United States were factors for illicit
drug use among the subjects. Furthermore, they concluded, "...women
have increased vulnerability compared with men" (Vega, et al., 1998, p.
1839).

Although these studies have found a link between language
preference and drug use, this is not to suggest that language preference
is a causal factor for deviant behavior, but rather is an indicator of an
individual's level of acculturation. In addition, these studies suggest that
the drug use problem among Puerto Ricans on the mainland, as with
other Hispanics, cannot be attributed to a general increase in drug use by
Puerto Ricans and others in their native cultures but to factors related to
the migration experience.

Researchers studying drug use among Hispanics, including Puerto
Ricans, have frequently suggested acculturation alone as the explanation
for drug use patterns of Hispanics in the United States. However, the
plausible alternative explanation that we are suggesting is that it is the

movement away from a traditional outlook itself, which had once served as a brake or control mechanism that effects an increase in drug use. As we will indicate through the data presented in Chapter 7, this loss of identification with one's tradition may have an impact even though there are no specific drug regulatory traditional norms.

ALCOHOL AND DRUG USE OUTCOME INDICATORS

In order to facilitate the analyses of the data four alcohol and drug outcome indices were created and are described below:

1. Index of levels of alcohol use
2. Index of extent of drinking in different settings
3. Index of number of drinking problems
4. Index of drug use

INDEX OF LEVELS OF ALCOHOL USE

Respondents were asked screening questions resulting in a classification of three groups: those who never drank, those who drank at some point in the past but not during the prior year, and those drinking during the past year. Less than half the women (47.2%) drank in the past year compared with two thirds of the men (67.7%). The literature on Hispanic drinking repeatedly shows that Hispanic men are much more likely than women to be drinkers, but this does not mean that all Puerto Rican males could be classified, even loosely, as a current drinker—only a little over half (55.6%) drank during the past year. Nearly twice as many women reported that they never drank (26.5% of women vs. 13.5% of men, $p < .001$).

Respondents were asked to determine the frequency and amount of recent use separately for beer, wine, and liquor. Of these beverages, beer

TABLE 4.1. Percent Using Each Beverage Recently by Gender

At least once	Male		Female		Total	
	N	%	N	%	N	%
Wine[a]	149	49.3	194	64.5	343	56.9
Beer[b]	268	88.7	217	72.1	485	80.4
Liquor[c]	191	63.2	170	56.5	361	59.9

[a] $\chi^2(1, N = 603) = 14.04, p < .001.$
[b] $\chi^2(1, N = 603) = 26.54, p < .001.$
[c] $\chi^2(1, N = 603) = 2.87, p > .05.$

was most likely to have been used, followed by liquor and then wine (80.4%, 59.9%, and 56.9%). There were significant differences between males and females in their choice of beverage with women more likely than men to choose wine and men more likely than women to choose beer and liquor (see Table 4.1).

In addition, a greater percentage of all drinkers reported more extensive drinking of beer (16.9% of all drinker reported drinking five or six cans of beer "nearly every time" or "more than half the time" when they drank beer) than five or six "drinks" of liquor (8.6%) or five or six glasses of wine (2.3%) (data not shown).

An index of alcohol use was developed separately for each of the beverages. Each index was created by combining information from three questions determining amount and frequency for each beverage type. Each question asked: "When you drink them (the beverage), how often do you have as many as five or six drinks?" This was repeated for three or four and one or two drinks. Those who stated that they had five or six drinks of the beverage "nearly every time" were assigned a weight of 4. Those who stated that they had five or six drinks "more than half the time" were assigned a weight of 3; "less than half" were assigned a 2; "once in a while" a 1; and "never" received a 0. For the remaining applicable cases of three or four drinks, the assignment was similar, as

was the case for one or two drinks. These questions were asked for the
higher amounts first. Respondents who said "nearly every time" or
"more than half the time" to the higher amounts in descending order
were not asked for the lower amounts. Therefore, comparable weights
were assigned to these skipped questions based on their responses to the
higher amounts.

TABLE 4.2. Level of Beverage Alcohol Use by Gender

	Male		Female		Total	
	N	%	N	%	N	%
Wine use[a]						
Low drinker	50	34.8	60	31.4	110	32.8
Moderate drinker	46	31.9	85	44.5	131	39.1
Heavy drinker	48	33.3	46	24.1	94	28.1
Total	144	100.0	191	100.0	335	100.0
Beer use[b]						
Low drinker	53	20.2	83	38.6	136	28.5
Moderate drinker	96	36.6	82	38.1	178	37.3
Heavy drinker	113	43.1	50	23.3	163	34.2
Total	262	100.0	215	100.0	477	100.0
Liquor use[c]						
Low drinker	62	33.9	70	41.7	132	37.6
Moderate drinker	47	25.7	66	39.3	113	32.2
Heavy drinker	74	40.4	32	19.0	106	30.2
Total	183	100.0	168	100.0	351	100.0

a $\chi^2(2, N = 335) = 6.09, p < .05.$
b $\chi^2(2, N = 477) = 27.71, p < .001.$
c $\chi^2(2, N = 351) = 19.72, p < .001.$

TABLE 4.3. Index of Level of Alcohol Use by Gender

	Male		Female		Total	
	N	%	N	%	N	%
Low drinker (score 1,2)	60	21.1	101	34.8	161	28.0
Moderate drinker (score 3,4)	104	36.6	102	35.2	206	35.9
Heavy drinker (score 5–9)	120	42.3	87	30.0	207	36.1
Total	284	100.0	290	100.0	574	100.0

$\chi^2(2, N = 574) = 15.66, p < .001$.

An additive index was created in this manner for all three beverage types. Each amount/frequency index was trichotomized into low, moderate, and heavy drinkers for each type. This is presented, indicating the differences between male and female drinking, in Table 4.2. For all three beverage types, males are more likely to be heavy drinkers (as defined by the index criteria) than females.

These three indices were combined into an index of level of alcohol use by adding the assigned scores of 1 = low drinker, 2 = moderate drinker, or 3 = heavy drinker (nonusers of the beverage were scored 0) for each of the three beverage categories and the resulting sum trichotomized. The created index shows that males are significantly more likely than females to be "heavy" drinkers. This is presented in Table 4.3.

INDEX OF EXTENT OF DRINKING IN DIFFERENT SETTINGS

As already noted above, the literature reports that drinking among Hispanic women is highly regulated. It also is suggested that when drinking does occur among women, it is more likely to happen within private settings (Aguirre-Molina, 1991; Fernandez-Pol, Bluestone, Missouri, Morales, & Mizruchi, 1986). While the number of different places at which one drinks does not by itself define a problem whether it is at home only or in many different settings, it does provide a degree of measure of the willingness that one has to expose one's self to drinking opportunities. While solitary drinkers (at home only) may be as much at risk (or perhaps even more so given the lack of community scrutiny) of becoming dependent on or habituated to alcohol, they are less likely to be exposed to the drinking-related problems that may arise in social situations, i.e., drinking outside of the home (e.g., bar brawls, drunken driving, quarrels with family members in public, etc.).

In order to examine the milieu in which respondents drink, they were asked questions regarding their drinking in various settings. The questions addressed how often they drank in eight different settings: during the evening with dinner at a restaurant; during lunch at restaurant; at clubs or organizational meetings; in bars, taverns, or cocktail lounges; at someone's home party; while spending quiet time at home; when a friend comes to visit; and when in the company of friends in public places such as parks, street, and parking lots. The responses available ranged between "never" (weighted with an assigned value of 1) to "almost all the time" (with a weighted value of 5). Table 4.4 presents the percentage of drinkers who attended each type of setting, and the frequency of drinking by the respondents when attending each setting.

Of the 603 persons in the sample who drank during the past year, there was considerable variation in the places in which they drank. Of those places cited, respondents were least likely to drink when they went out for lunch (90.2% said never or less than half the time) and most likely to drink at a bar (73.3% cited "about half the time" or more frequently) and at a party (60.2% responded similarly). For all locations, women drank less often than men did. This was found to be significant for dining at restaurants, drinking at parties, drinking at home, and street drinking. Men reported drinking at a significantly higher number of places than women, 3.44 versus 2.92 ($t = 3.44$, df = 509, $p < .001$).

TABLE 4.4. Percent of Current Drinkers Attending Each Setting and
Frequency of Drinking at Settings by Gender

How often do you have a drink when you...	Male		Female		Total	
	N	%	N	%	N	%
1. Go out for an evening meal in a restaurant						
Percent of drinkers	199	66.8	211	72.0	410	69.3
Never	66	33.2	69	32.7	135	32.9
Less than half the time	44	22.1	77	36.5	121	29.5
About half the time	21	10.6	29	13.7	50	12.2
More than half the time	19	9.5	15	7.1	34	8.3
Almost all the time	49	24.6	21	10.0	70	17.1
Total	199	100.0	211	100.0	410	100.0

$\chi^2(4, N = 410) = 21.68, p < .001$.

How often do you have a drink when you...	Male		Female		Total	
2. Go out for lunch in a restaurant						
Percent of drinkers	132	44.3	122	41.6	254	43.0
Never	83	62.9	91	74.6	174	68.5
Less than half the time	32	24.2	23	18.9	55	21.7
About half the time	7	5.3	4	3.3	11	4.3
More than half the time	2	1.5	1	.8	3	1.2
Almost all the time	8	6.1	3	2.5	11	4.3
Total	132	100.0	122	100.0	254	100.0

$\chi^2(4, N = 254) = 4.87, p > .05$.

How often do you have a drink when you...	Male		Female		Total	
3. Go to club or organizational meetings						
Percent of drinkers	84	28.2	71	24.2	155	26.2
Never	25	29.8	30	72.3	55	35.5
Less than half the time	18	21.4	15	21.1	33	21.3
About half the time	18	21.4	9	12.7	27	17.4
More than half the time	6	7.1	6	8.5	12	7.7
Almost all the time	17	20.2	11	15.5	28	18.1
Total	84	100.0	71	100.0	155	100.0

$\chi^2(4, N = 155) = 3.95, p > .05$.

4. Go to bars, taverns or cocktail lounges

Percent of drinkers	95	31.9	55	18.8	150	25.3
Never	7	7.4	6	10.9	13	8.7
Less than half the time	15	15.8	12	21.8	12	18.0
About half the time	10	10.5	7	12.7	17	11.3
More than half the time	15	15.8	7	12.7	22	14.7
Almost all the time	48	50.5	23	41.8	71	47.3
Total	95	100.0	55	100.0	150	100.0

$\chi^2(4, N = 150) = 2.13, p > .05.$

5. Go to a party in someone else's home

Percent of drinkers	214	72.0	218	74.4	432	73.1
Never	28	13.1	29	13.3	57	13.2
Less than half the time	45	21.0	70	32.1	115	26.6
About half the time	28	13.1	32	14.7	60	13.9
More than half the time	31	14.5	36	16.5	67	15.5
Almost all the time	82	38.3	51	23.4	133	30.8
Total	214	100.0	218	100.0	432	100.0

$\chi^2(4, N = 432) = 13.28, p < .01.$

6. Spend a quiet evening at home

Percent of drinkers	287	96.3	276	94.2	563	94.8
Never	134	46.7	165	59.8	299	53.1
Less than half the time	59	20.6	59	21.4	118	21.0
About half the time	33	11.5	23	8.3	56	9.9
More than half the time	31	10.8	9	3.3	40	7.1
Almost all the time	30	10.5	20	7.2	50	8.9
Total	287	100.0	276	100.0	563	100.0

$\chi^2(4, N = 563) = 18.89, p < .001.$

7. Have friends drop over and visit in your house

Percent of drinkers	186	62.4	195	66.6	381	64.5
Never	61	32.8	73	37.4	134	35.2
Less than half the time	53	28.5	65	33.3	118	31.0
About half the time	27	14.5	24	12.3	51	13.4
More than half the time	18	9.7	18	9.2	36	9.4
Almost all the time	27	14.5	15	7.7	42	11.0
Total	186	100.0	195	100.0	381	100.0

$\chi^2(4, N = 381) = 5.69, p > .05.$

8. Hang around with friends in a public place such as a park, street or parking lot

Percent of drinkers	159	53.4	92	31.4	251	42.5
Never	55	34.6	51	55.4	106	42.2
Less than half the time	36	22.6	32	34.8	68	27.1
About half the time	17	10.7	3	3.3	20	8.0
More than half the time	15	9.4	1	1.1	16	6.4
Almost all the time	36	22.6	5	5.4	41	16.3
Total	159	100.0	92	100.0	251	100.0

$\chi^2(4, N = 251) = 30.13, p < .001.$

An index of extent of drinking in different settings was created by adding the responses to the items presented in Table 4.4. A response of "never" was assigned a value of 1 and "almost all of the time" was assigned a value of 5. Missing information for any variable was replaced by the average of all available responses for that case. The trichotomized index is presented in Table 4.5. As shown, males not only were more likely to drink in a greater variety of settings than women, but they also were almost twice as likely to drink more heavily than women in the different settings (43.7% vs. 22.2%, $p < .001$).

TABLE 4.5.   Index of Extent of Drinking in Different Settings by Gender

	Male		Female		Total	
Score	N	%	N	%	N	%
Low (score 9–12)	85	32.3	112	45.2	197	38.6
Med (score 13–16)	63	24.0	81	32.7	144	28.2
High (score 17–36)	115	43.7	55	22.2	170	33.3
Total*	263	100.0	248	100.0	511	100.0

$\chi^2(2, N = 511) = 26.71, p < .001.$

* Excluding Abstainers and 92 drinkers with missing information for all settings.

INDEX OF NUMBER OF DRINKING PROBLEMS

Respondents who drank during the past year and those who ever drank more than seven drinks at one time but did not drink during past year ($N = 35$) were read a list of possible "experiences" they may have had "in connection with drinking." These experiences (a total of 35) consisted of problems in the areas of family and social interactions, employment, health, loss of control over drinking, and antisocial behavior. A simple additive index was created for each area. The percent of drinkers who cited each item as well as the percentage for each index is presented in Table 4.6.

It is striking to note that in every instance men are more likely than women are to report a problem. When examining the grouped categories we find that males are 9.2 times as likely to cite an employment problem than are women, followed by family and social problems (4 times as likely), antisocial behavior (3.4 times as likely), health (2.7 times as likely), and loss of control (2.3 times as likely). All grouped differences were significant at the .001 level. The most often cited problem for men was "skipping meals while drinking" (27.9%) followed closely by "blackout of previous nights drinking" (26,4%) For women, it was "blackouts" (11.7%) followed by "skipping meals" (10.7%).

TABLE 4.6. Percent of Drinkers Indicating Ever Had Alcohol Related
Problems

Problem area	Male	Female	Total
Family & social (at least 1 problem)	29.2	7.3	18.9***
Drinking interfered with spare time activities	15.2	1.7	8.9***
Spouse angry about my drinking	22.2	3.1	13.3***
Spouse threatened to leave because of drinking	10.7	1.4	6.3***
Family and friends pressure to curtail drinking	15.2	3.4	9.7***
Employment (at least 1 problem)	9.2	1.0	5.3***
Lost job or nearly lost job because of drinking	4.6	0.7	2.8**
Fellow workers pressure to curtail drinking	7.3	—	3.9***
Drinking hurt promotions, raises, or better job	2.7	0.3	1.6*
Health (at least 1 problem)	38.1	14.3	26.9***
Skipped meals while drinking	27.9	10.7	19.8***
Hands shook on morning after drinking	12.1	4.1	8.4***
Nighttime sweats due to drinking	7.9	2.4	5.3**
Drinking-related illness prevented normal work	10.3	3.5	7.1***
Believed drinking was seriously affecting health	15.8	6.2	11.3***
Physician suggested drinking curtailment	15.8	5.9	11.2***
Fits or seizures after cessation of drinking	4.6	1.0	2.9**
DTs after cessation	4.0	1.0	2.6*
Saw or heard things not there after curtailment	4.0	0.7	2.4**
Loss of control over drinking (at least 1 problem)	41.4	18.0	30.3***
Often drink first thing after waking up	10.0	2.7	6.6***
Taken strong drink in morning for hangover	13.3	3.1	8.5***
Blackout of previous night's drinking	26.4	11.7	19.5***
Need more alcohol for same effects	12.7	2.1	7.7***
Obsessive need for a drink	9.7	2.7	6.4***
Stayed intoxicated for several days at a time	10.0	1.4	6.0***
Once began drinking, continued until intoxicated	14.2	3.8	9.4***

Continued drinking after promising self not to	21.3	5.2	13.8***
Try to cut down but was unable	15.5	3.8	10.0***
Afraid I was an alcoholic	12.5	4.8	8.9***
Drinking 5+ at a sitting at least once a week	25.2	9.3	17.7***
Felt drinking was not under my control	15.0	4.8	10.2***
Antisocial behavior (at least 1 problem)	23.8	7.0	15.9***
Heated arguments while drinking	18.8	5.5	12.6***
Fights while drinking	11.5	4.5	8.2***
Police officer questioned or warned about drinking	6.1	0.7	3.6***
Drinking led to me hurt in car or other accident	5.2	1.0	3.2**
Drinking led to others hurt or property damage	1.8	1.0	1.5
Nonautomobile trouble with law due to drink	3.6	1.4	2.6
Arrested as DUI	2.7	0.3	1.6*
Total number of drinkers	336	300	638

$* p < .05; \quad ** p < .01; \quad *** p < .001.$

An index of number of drinking problems was created by counting the number of family, employment, health, loss of control over drinking, and antisocial behavior problems the respondents ever had. While some students of alcoholism may extrapolate from certain of these responses (especially the "loss of control" items) and suggest that an index of alcoholism could be constructed based on similarities to currently used alcoholism screening tests, this not only is beyond the scope of this volume but would digress into the controversy of problem drinking versus the disease (alcohol addiction) concept of alcoholism. Some of these drinkers may be alcohol addicts by any definition, but from the traditional Puerto Rican social definition there is little if any distinction for example between the *borrachona* (a female drunk) and the woman engaged in nonnormative drinking. Similarly, little distinction exists between the "alcoholic" and the "drunk." In addition, we do not wish to

TABLE 4.7. Index of Number of Drinking Problems by Gender

	Male		Female		Total	
	N	%	N	%	N	%
None[a]	158	46.6	227	75.8	385	60.3
One	44	13.0	28	9.4	72	11.4
2-6	64	18.9	25	8.4	89	13.9
7 or more	73	21.5	19	6.4	92	14.4
Total	339	100.0	299	100.0	638	100.0

$\chi^2(3, N = 638) = 62.44, p < .001.$
[a] Excluding abstainers.

promote an impression that a greater number of problems is more indicative of the disease concept of alcoholism than of a more general notion of problem drinking (Jellinek, 1960).

The number of problems reported by the respondents ranged between 0 and 32 and is presented in Table 4.7. Nearly 40% of the drinkers reported having at least one problem caused by alcohol in their lifetime. Males reported an average of four times as many problems as females (M = 4.28 vs. 1.14, t = 6.91, df = 636, p < .001).

INDEX OF DRUG USE

Goode (1989) has taken the position that mood or mind altering drugs are "both chemical substances and social, cultural and symbolic phenomena that are perceived, dealt with, and used in certain ways by the general society and by groups within it" (p. 38). From this perspective drugs are more than just chemicals, they also are whatever societies or groups define them to be: good or evil. Alcohol obviously can be included in Goode's conception. As stated earlier, certain benefits are ascribed to alcohol use (e.g., individual relaxation, social lubricant, and group bonding); nevertheless, other drugs (particularly in the

United States) are not perceived or dealt with so benignly. As Goode (1989) states,

> ...the most widely accepted general approach to drug use and abuse...cannot be located in any particular field. It is adhered to by much, probably most, of the public, and by most practitioners....It is called the *medical* or the *pathology* model, and its basic assumption is that nonmedical drug use is very much like a disease—a malfunctioning, an abnormality, a pathology. It is not "normal" to use drugs outside a medical context, only a drug-free existence is normal. (p. 54)

Although in the Hispanic culture there is no specific traditional condemnation of drug use, as with alcohol, its use by women can jeopardize the values defined by the concept of *marianismo*. It is plausible to assume that therefore, drugs are implicitly prohibited for women by the same traditional norms as alcohol. For men, however, the issue of illegality and a general lack of social approbation must suffice.

While the main focus of the data used in this study was to examine patterns of alcohol use, there were a limited number of questions on drugs. All the respondents (regardless of their alcohol use) were asked questions related to drug use. They were asked whether they had used different substances, i.e., uppers (including cocaine), downers (including Valium), codeine or methadone, marijuana, hallucinogens, and heroin during the 12 months prior to the interview, but not whether they had used the drugs before then. Therefore, this study will not be able to report or examine findings for those who had ever used drugs, but only on the more current users. Table 4.8 presents the percent of individuals reporting use of the specific drug during the past year.

Men were more likely to have used these drugs than the women were, with the difference in use significant for uppers, codeine, and marijuana. For both men and women, marijuana was found to be the prevailing drug used during the 12 months prior to the interview. In their 1986 *Statewide Household Survey of Substance Abuse* report of more

TABLE 4.8. Percent Indicating Drugs Used during Prior 12 Months by
Gender

Drug	Male	Female	Total
Uppers (speed, amphetamines, or cocaine)	4.9	1.9	3.1**
Downers (tranquilizers, barbiturates, Quaaludes, Librium, or Valium)	2.5	2.2	2.3
Codeine or methadone	2.2	0.8	1.4*
Marijuana, hash, THC or grass	10.1	3.3	6.1***
Hallucinogens (LSD, PCP, mescaline, psilocybin)	0.2	—	0.1
Heroin or opium	0.2	—	0.1
Total N	446	638	1084

$*p < .05;$ $**p < .01;$ $***p < .001.$

than 6300 residents, the New York State Division of Substance Abuse Service also found that marijuana was the "leading illicit drug used by both Hispanic and nonHispanic residents in New York State" (Frank, Schmeidler, Marel, & Maranda, 1988, p. 4)

An additive index of drug use was created and dichotomized. Approximately 10% of the respondents reported using at least one of the stated substances during the past year with men more than twice as likely as women (14.3% vs. 6.6%, $p < .001$). It again should be stressed that this is a representative community sample but does not include youths under the age of 18.

CORRELATIONS BETWEEN OUTCOME MEASURES

Correlations of the three alcohol indices and drug use are presented in Table 4.9. All these indices are significantly related with the highest correlation found between recent levels of alcohol use and extent of drinking in different settings. The lowest correlation is between number of drinking problems and drug use. Many persons in the addictions

TABLE 4.9.   Correlations between Outcome Variables

(N = 578)

Outcome variable	2	3	4
Index of levels of alcohol use	.39***	.22***	.13**
Index of extent of drinking in different settings		.22***	.19***
Index of number of drinking problems			.10*
Index of drug use			

* p < .05;   ** p < .01;   *** p < .001.

industry in the United States continue to press the notion of "dual addiction" not as a rarity but as a commonplace. Our data do not support this. Even using the very liberal definition of problem drinking as one or more problems and using *any* drug use as criteria, the correlation may be surprisingly low to some of those who would have it otherwise.

BACKGROUND VARIABLES AND SUBSTANCE USE OUTCOMES

We have examined how gender is related to drinking and drug use outcomes. How is age, place of birth, time in United States, ethnic identity, and education related to outcomes? Other considerations such as the importance of religiosity and fatalism may very possibly influence substance use status and history and will be analyzed in Chapter 6.

Younger Puerto Rican men and women are more likely to be drinkers and drug users. For males, having drinking problems increases with age, while for women age is negatively related to level of drinking but not related to problems. Being born in the United States increases the likelihood of becoming a drinker and a drug user for both males and

TABLE 4.10. Correlations between Background Variables and Substance Use
Outcomes for Males and Females[a]

Outcome	Age	Place of birth	Ethnic identify	Education
Males				
Drinker	-.18***	.18***	-.05	.17***
Level of Drinking	-.07	.06	-.02	.10
Extent of drinking in different settings	-.08	.15*	.16**	.14*
Number of drinking problems	.23***	-.22***	-.08	-.22***
Drug use	-.26***	.25***	.12**	.21***
Females				
Drinker	-.29***	.20***	.16***	.23***
Level of drinking	-.14*	.05	.06	.04
Extent of drinking in different settings	.01	.02	.06	.13*
Number of drinking problems	.03	.02	-.01	-.06
Drug use	-.15***	.14***	.14***	.12**

[a] N for drinker and drug use: males = 445, females = 638;
N for remaining variables: males = 284, females = 290.
* $p < .05$ ** $p < .01$ *** $p < .001$.

females. For males, it also increased the likelihood of drinking in a variety of settings, but being born in the United States correlated negatively with the number of drinking problems that emerge ($r = -.22$). This suggests that those Puerto Rican males born in the United States may learn to drink more in conformity with the Anglo norms, thus appearing to have fewer problems. A weaker ethnic identification with being Puerto Rican was found to increase the extent of drinking indifferent settings as well as the likelihood of being a drug user for men, while for women it increased their likelihood of being a drinker and the likelihood of being a drug user. Higher levels of education also were found to increase the likelihood of being a drinker, the extent of drinking, and the likelihood of being a drug user, but among males education reduced the likelihood of problematic drinking.

CHAPTER 5

DRINKING ATTITUDES AND BELIEFS

How do parents' drinking affect the likelihood of their children drinking? What are the expectations of the effect of drinking for one's self and for others? What are the perceived benefits of drinking by men and women? What is the relationship between alcohol expectancies and abstinence, level of drinking, and problematic outcomes? What rationales are used for drinking and which ones are used to curb ones' drinking? Do positive attitudes encourage drinking and do negative attitudes discourage drinking? What are the Puerto Rican norms concerning how much to drink and where? How much permission is given for persons to drink at different ages? How do Puerto Ricans view alcoholism and drunkenness? Who goes for help and where?

Alcohol consumption in this society, as in most, is vested with many different and sometimes conflicting attitudes and beliefs as to the legitimacy of use as well as consequences. These beliefs may be institutionalized, as in the ritual use of alcohol in religious ceremonies and sacraments, societal laws restricting consumption by minors, or reflect safety concerns as in driving under the influence legislation. In addition, alcohol beliefs and attitudes may be loosely institutionalized in secular accompaniments to important occasions such as wedding and *bar mitzvah* parties, baptism of children, and holidays. Many of these attitudes and beliefs are generationally linked and may invoke the collective traditional system of beliefs and attitudes of one's religion or ethnicity. These often will vary from one group to another.

Because of societal concerns to prevent problems of alcohol and drug abuse in both the Hispanic and Anglo communities, efforts at changing attitudes in the hopes of altering or preventing undesired behaviors appear to have become routine. Organizations such as MADD. (Mothers Against Drunk Driving) and DARE (Drug Abuse Resistance Education) are national and their messages reach millions. In addition to deliberate societal intervention in the manipulation and formation of attitudes is the fact that most people in the Hispanic and Anglo communities have grown up with sets of attitudes that already are part of their ethnic cultural heritages and have seen and received attitudinal messages concerning alcohol and substance use directly from their parents. In the Hispanic communities, as in this study of a Puerto Rican mainland community, there are strong and often consistent attitudes concerning alcohol that have been known for generations. However, no such clarity exists for other substance misuse that society has deemed illicit; therefore, in this chapter we shall examine Puerto Rican attitudes concerning alcohol use only.

TABLE 5.1. Percent of Abstinent Parents by Abstinent Respondents

	Both parents present and abstinent	All others
Abstinent respondents	43.1%	14.9%
All others	56.9%	85.1%
Total N	239	845

$\chi^2(1, N = 1084) = 88.82, p < .001.$

FAMILY ROLE MODELS

For Puerto Ricans, as in all other ethnic groups, the family is the first line of attitude formation concerning drinking. At what age one is old enough to drink, how much to drink, what to drink, and many other questions are answered directly or informally by what children pick up in familial situations. In addition, children not only hear what is said about alcohol use, they observe parental drinking behavior.

Questions were asked concerning the respondent's mother and father to determine if abstinent respondents were living in homes with abstinent parents when they were about 16 years of age (see Table 5.1). Table 5.1 supports what many believe to be a commonsense point of view: abstinent parents are more likely to raise children who also will be abstinent than are drinking parents. Modeling theory suggests that mothers are the significant role models for their daughters as are fathers for their sons. With regard to offspring drinking, we would expect that a father's abstinent behavior would have a higher correlation with his son's abstinence and a daughter with her mother's abstinence. This indeed is the case as borne out by Table 5.2, but the father's abstinence seems more important even to his daughter than the mother–daughter relationship.

TABLE 5.2. Correlations of Parental Abstainers by Respondent Abstainers

	Abstinent fathers	Abstinent mothers
Male abstainers	.20[a]***	.12[b]*
Female abstainers	.34[c]**	.26[d]***

[a]$N = 367$; [b]$N = 526$; [c]$N = 430$; [d]$N = 621$.
*$p < .05$; **$p < .01$; ***$p < .001$.

Having a mother who was present and abstinent until the
respondent was 16 years of age appears to be less significant for
offspring abstinence than having a father present and abstinent for both
male and female respondents. Even mere parental disapproval of adult
drinking during the respondents' formative years appears to be
positively correlated with later drinking curtailment, as seen in Table 5.3.

When we compare Tables 5.2 and 5.3, parental disapproval of adult
drinking does not appear as important as does parental abstinence, with
the exception of the mother–son relationship. However, since abstinence
may be a personal choice or the effect of a particular religious affiliation,
a parent's abstinent behavior may not have reflected his or her attitudes
about the correctness of drinking by others outside the family. In Table
5.4, we present the effect of parents who are both abstinent and
disapproving of adult drinking upon their children's later drinking.

TABLE 5.3. Correlations of Parental Disapproval of Adult Drinking by
Respondent Abstainers

	Disapproving fathers	Disapproving mothers
Male abstainers	.10[a]**	.16[b]***
Female abstainers	.21[c]***	.17[d]***

[a]$N = 369$; [b]$N = 528$; [c]$N = 431$; [d]$N = 623$.
*$p < .05$; **$p < .01$; ***$p < .001$.

TABLE 5.4. Correlations of Parental Abstinence and Disapproval of Adult
Drinking by Respondent Abstinence

	Abstinent and disapproving fathers	Abstinent and disapproving mothers
Male abstainers	.20[a]***	.14[b]**
Female abstainers	.34[c]***	.26[d]***

[a]$N = 369$;   [b]$N = 528$;   [c]$N = 431$;   [d]$N = 623$.

*$p < .05$;   **$p < .01$;   ***$p < .001$.

When we compare Table 5.2 to Table 5.4, we find that with the exception of the mother–son relationship, nothing is gained by the element of disapproval being added to having abstinent parents. It appears that disapproval is not as significant as behavior in influencing later drinking practices of children. But what about contradictory messages? If we examine the influence of parents who were inconsistent, that is, disapproving of drinking for others but not themselves abstinent, we find that (again with the exception of the mother–son relationship) inconsistent parents have the lowest correlation rates with offspring abstinence (see Table 5.5).

Why are there consistent exceptions of the disapproving mother and abstinent son relationships in Tables 5.3 to 5.5? One possible explanation is that in the Puerto Rican family, as in other Hispanic and ethnic groups, male children are the pride and center of parental attention. Mothers often fawn over and cuddle the male child, who in turn reveres the mother. The indulgence of the Puerto Rican mother for the minor misdeeds of the male child (compared to the daughter from whom greater subservience is expected) heightens the importance of maternal disapproval when it does occur.

TABLE 5.5. Correlations of Parental Drinking and Disapproval of Adult
Drinking by Respondent Abstinence

	Drinking and disapproving fathers	Drinking and disapproving mothers
Male abstainers	.09[a]	.17[b]***
Female abstainers	.21[c]***	.17[d]***

[a]N = 369;   [b]N = 528;   [c]N = 431;   [d]N = 623.
*p < .05;   **p < .01;   ***p < .001.

In a practical sense, the findings in Tables 5.1 to 5.5 suggest that the "just say no" message of preaching to young persons to prevent alcohol use, drug use, cigarette smoking, and nonmarital sex may have little if any impact when parental behavior is not consistent with preachment. Even though parents may not be using illicit drugs, the paradigm of many if not most adults using legal pills or alcohol to "feel good" (whether through the absence of pain or pursuit of pleasure/relaxation) is not easy to rationalize in a manner reasonable enough to prevent young persons from making the same associations. If responsible drinking for pleasure is reasonable for adults, then it may appear that it is reasonable for a young person who believes he or she is choosing a responsible set of behavioral acts. Similarly, if chemicals can produce a desired positive effect when taken responsibly, it is difficult to argue than mere illegality rather than intrinsic merits of the effect of the chemicals ingested should preclude responsible choices.

DRINKING EXPECTANCIES

Community-held attitudes regarding the use of a substance have been found to have an affect on how that substance is used (Peele, 1989; Pittman, 1967; Weil, 1986). As indicated in the previous chapter, Pittman (1967) categorized cultures according to their attitude toward drinking—attitudes that serve to control the drinking of individuals in each culture. Andrew Weil (1986) in his discussions of drug use argues that the ritualistic way in which substances are used in some cultures is an important factor regarding the low levels of problems attributed to use of drugs or alcohol for them. Furthermore, Weil argues that drugs in these cultures are not taken as a response to a problem or stressful situation but are part and parcel of cultural expectations. Along the same lines, Peele (1985) states "social-learning theorists have been especially active in alcoholism, where they have analyzed how alcoholics' expectations and beliefs about what alcohol will do for them influence the rewards and behaviors associated with drinking" (p. 70). This effect had been presented in a slightly different form a decade earlier by Weil in his consideration of the impact of set and setting:

> Set is a person's expectations of what a drug will do to him, considered in the context of his whole personality. Setting is the environment, both physical and social, in which a drug is taken.... (T)he combined effects of set and setting can easily overshadow the pharmacological effects of a drug... (Weil, 1986, p. 29)

Although Weil was referring in this paragraph more specifically to psychedelic drugs, many drinkers are aware that their expectations and social situation while drinking often determines the effect of the ingestion of alcohol. For example, readers who are drinkers will know that the effect of drinking several cocktails in a relatively short period of time at a cocktail party often seems to heighten the excitement of the situation and loosen inhibitions, while the same amount of alcohol in the same time period when one is alone at home is more likely to produce a calming relaxed state, if not a soporific condition. The attitudes and expectations that one holds regarding drinking and the possible rewards then are an important component in the examination of drinking habits and problems of the participants in this study.

Expectancies, as with the older concept of attitudes, are predispositions to act in a predictable manner given a defined set of situational determinants. In this sense, we may say that attitudes can predict behavior given knowledge of the group from which they were derived. Some studies have indicated that expectancies may help predict drinking outcomes among Hispanics (Cervantes, Gilbert, Snyder, & Padilla, 1990–1991; Marin, 1996; Velez-Blasini, 1997).

EXPECTANCIES ABOUT DRINKING BY OTHERS

All respondents in this study were asked to rate how strongly they agreed or disagreed with general statements regarding "how you think most men and women feel when they drink." Table 5.6 presents the percent of individuals who stated they "strongly agree" and "agree" with each possible effect.

When comparing abstainers to drinkers, we find that while there are no significant differences between male and female abstainers for any of the items, there are differences for a number of items between male and female drinkers (items 2, 4, 6, 8, 11, 12, and 13). We find that female drinkers regard the influence of alcohol on male behavior to be mainly negative. They were more likely than male drinkers to view alcohol as increasing *male* likelihood of getting into fights, feeling more depressed, feeling out of control, and acting against their moral principles (items 2, 4, 6, 8). The negative expectancies held by women regarding male drinking likely reflect the experiences of women in a culture where they are not uncommonly the victims (psychological and physical) of the male drinkers in their families as they grow up, as well as when they get married and form their own households.

On the other hand, female drinkers expected that alcohol would have a negative effect on women more related to internal conditions (depression and guilt) than behavioral. This probably reflects the awareness that social control norms are effective in governing and limiting the alcohol behavior of women and that women who drink

TABLE 5.6. Percent of Drinkers Stating They Agree or Strongly Agree with Each Drinking Result by Gender

	Abstainers		Drinkers	
	Male	Female	Male	Female
Expectations	$N = 148$	$N = 345$	$N = 284$	$N = 290$
1. Most men have more fun when they drink	41.2	46.4	64.4	63.8
2. Most men get into more fights when they drink	96.6	94.2	86.2	93.1**
3. Most men feel more friendly and less shy after a few drinks	68.2	73.8	83.1	84.5
4. Most men feel more depressed when they drink	56.8	59.2	41.9	50.5*
5. Most men feel guilty when they drink	50.3	57.5	44.9	51.6
6. Most men feel out of control after a few drinks	91.2	92.5	73.6	82.4**
7. Most men become more interested in sex after a few drinks	60.5	64.1	65.0	74.6*
8. Most men are more likely to go against their moral principles after a few drinks	92.6	94.7	85.9	92.7**
9. Most women have more fun when they drink	55.8	52.0	74.6	71.0
10. Most women get into more fights when they drink	83.7	76.5	60.7	60.3
11. Most women feel more friendly and less shy after a few drinks	78.2	78.7	92.3	86.1*
12. Most women feel more depressed when they drink	57.5	63.6	41.6	56.3***
13. Most women feel guilty when they drink	54.8	57.3	40.4	54.2***
14. Most women feel out of control after a few drinks.	89.2	91.0	76.3	76.7
15. Most women become more interested in sex after a few drinks	58.9	63.7	70.8	64.2
16. Most women are more likely to go against their moral principles after a few drinks	89.2	90.7	82.1	80.9

* $p < .05$ ** $p < .01$ *** $p < .001$.

are morally wrong. We also found that, with the exception of the expectations of depression, guilt, and loss of inhibitions (items 11, 12, and 13) the percentage of males and females agreeing with statements when the drinker was female were very similar.

When we combine males and females (data not shown) we find that there are considerable differences between the combined abstainers and combined drinkers. In all but one item (15), there are statistically significant differences between abstainers and drinkers with the abstainers being more negative for each item.

This much more negative set of expectancies concerning the effects of drinking by abstainers is not unexpected. Many persons in societies that permit drinking have decided for varying reasons to discontinue their drinking; some for religious reasons, others for health, and still others because of problems with alcohol. In societies where drinking is the norm, pressure is often exerted on nondrinkers, even recovering alcoholics, to "have just one little drink." To resist these pressures, abstainers often need a set of reinforcing beliefs to help resist these social expectations in many different situations. Also, experiences of the authors in working with many recovering alcoholics and substance abusers who have gone through 12-step programs, therapeutic communities, and other resocialization/rehabilitation programs, have shown that participants often develop a cohesive belief and set of attitudes reflecting organizational or institutional ideology. We also have observed that they communicate these notions frequently to others likely to be sympathetic for what appears to be a means of feedback reinforcement. While this may be of great benefit in helping the recovery process, researchers have to be alert to this often retrospective alteration of attitudes and beliefs concerning substance use.

A further caveat regarding analysis of attitudinal variables: There is great value in determining predictive results, if at all possible, of any attitudes that may in turn affect behavior. However, there always is the problem of which came first. Even though abstainers may have many more negative attitudes concerning alcohol than drinkers, it is difficult if not impossible to determine in a cross-sectional rather than longitudinal survey the direction of association other than relying on good theoretical assumptions and more often the researchers much maligned common sense.

The expectancy statements were submitted to factor analysis principal component with varimax rotation. Four factors were distinguished: loss of control (loadings between .71879 and .61138), guilt and depression (between .79237 and .72899), increased fun (between .74549 and .64345), and increased sexual interest (between .83874 and .78189). Indices were created by counting the number of times a respondent "agreed" or "strongly agreed" with the expectancy statements in each area. The index of loss of control consisted of statements 2, 6, 8, 10, 14, and 16; an index of guilt feelings consisted of statements 4, 5, 12, and 13; the index of increased fun was composed of statements 1, 3, 9, and 11; and an index of increased sexual interest was created with statements 7 and 15. Cronbach's alpha reliability tests were .71 for loss of control, .77 for feelings of guilt and depression, .59 for increased fun, and .60 for increased sexual interest.

What is the relation, if any, between these four types of general expectations and abstinence, levels of drinking, and number of drinking problems for men and women? Correlations are presented in Table 5.7. We find that greater general expectations of loss of control as well as greater expectations of guilt and depression are related to greater likelihood of abstinence for the entire sample and lower levels of drinking among the drinkers group. In addition, greater expectations of increased fun were found to be related to the likelihood of being a drinker rather than an abstainer, as well as with higher levels of drinking among the drinkers. The strength of these relationships was similar for both men and women with the exception of the relationship between

TABLE 5.7. Correlations Between General Expectancy Factors and Outcome
Variables by Gender

General expectancy factors	Abstinent/drinker	Level of drinking	Number of drinking problems
Males	(N=432)	(N=284)	(N=339)
Loss of control	-.26***	-.16**	.13*
Guilt and depression	-.15**	-.16**	.17**
Increased fun	.28***	.14**	.00
Increased sexual interest	.08	.06	.05
Females	(N=635)	(N=290)	(N=299)
Loss of control	-.21***	-.12*	-.01
Guilt and depression	-.08*	-.28***	.10
Increased fun	.23***	.15**	-.01
Increased sexual interest	.07	.05	.04

* $p < .05$;   ** $p < .01$;   *** $p < .001$.

expectancies of guilt and depression and level of drinking among
women (-.28 for women compared to -.16 for men). This higher
expectation of guilt and depression as one drinks more may reflect the
cultural norms that tend to control female drinking through the instilling
of responsibility in women to maintain sobriety for the sake of the family
and children.

The relationship between negative expectancies (loss of control and
guilt and depression) and alcohol problems confronts those assuming
that negative attitudes may prevent alcohol-related problems. We found
that as the level of negative expectations increased, so did number of
problems, particularly among males. In this instance, it is just as
reasonable to assume that the negative expectancies were shaped by the
experience of alcohol problems rather than the opposite.

EXPECTED BENEFITS OF SELF DRINKING

Respondents who drank during the year prior to their interview were asked questions that tapped their perceptions of the benefits to them of using alcohol. The nine questions referred to drinking "after a hard day's work" in order to relax; drinking to "feel freer" and "do whatever I want"; drinking when "sad or depressed...(to) lift my spirits"; drinking to "help make sex more enjoyable"; drinking if "nervous or worried"; drinking to make "parties more fun"; drinking to make it "easier to talk to people"; drinking to be able to "discuss or argue a point more forcefully"; and drinking to "forget bad feelings." In one sense, these items reflect the more functional aspects of drinking compared with the more emotional and affect-related tone of items in Table 5.6. Available responses varied between "never" (with an assigned value of 0) and "always" (with an assigned value of 4).

Table 5.8 presents the percent of respondents citing that they received the specific benefit from drinking "always" or "almost always" by gender. As shown in Table 5.8 males are more likely than females to expect benefits from drinking in all nine possible benefit types (seven were significant). Do the perceived benefits relate to level of alcohol use and number of consequent alcohol problems? We found that the association between perceived benefits and drinking level for males (.32, $p < .001$) is somewhat higher than for females (.28, $p < .001$) and the relationship between perceived benefits and number of drinking problems also was stronger for males (.54, $p < .001$) than females (.40, $p < .001$). Alcohol appears to be viewed by men more than by women as beneficial to them, that is, as a problem solver in stressful situations (to relieve stress, to facilitate socializing, and for sexual enhancement). This use of alcohol as a problem solver and stress reducer has its dangers, as workers in the field of alcoholism treatment are well aware. The problem stems from the fact that alcohol is very effective in many of these stress-related situations and the more that one perceives and expects alcohol to work, uses the alcohol in this manner, and receives the gratification of success, the stronger the belief and expectation that it will be functional in future similar situations. This continuing reinforcement without traditional or ritualistic control and brakes runs the risk of alcohol becoming the response of choice to the stress-induced "flight or fight syndrome," with dependency becoming a very real possibility (Benson, 1975; Lieberman, 1987; Weil, 1986).

TABLE 5.8. Percent of Respondents Citing Always and Almost Always for Each Expected Benefit from Drinking by Gender

Expected Benefit	Male (N = 284)	Female (N = 290)	Total (N = 574)
1. After a hard day's work, a drink or two helps me to relax	17.3	2.4	9.8***
2. When I'm drinking, I feel freer to be myself and do whatever I want	13.0	7.6	10.3*
3. When I'm sad or depressed about the way things are going, a drink or two helps lift my spirits	16.5	8.3	12.4**
4. A drink or two can help make sex more enjoyable	9.2	2.8	5.9**
5. If I'm nervous or worried about something, a drink or two helps me relax	16.6	7.9	12.2**
6. Parties or get togethers are more fun when drinks are available	43.8	20.8	32.2***
7. If I have a couple of drinks, it's easier to talk to people	26.8	13.1	19.9***
8. I can discuss or argue a point more forcefully after I have had a drink or two	14.8	10.0	12.4
9. Alcohol makes it easier to forget bad feelings	12.0	8.6	10.3
Mean	1.69	0.81	$t = 5.60$***

* $p < .05$;   ** $p < .01$;   *** $p < .001$.

RATIONALES

Rather than the perceived and somewhat specific benefits of expectations, rationales are more general "excuses," often part of cultural truisms that one may offer as reasons for drinking or not drinking.

DRINKING RATIONALES

Do positive attitudes encourage extensive drinking? (Or possibly do people who drink more develop more excuses to drink?) Respondents were asked eight questions regarding how important each item was for their own drinking. The responses ranged from "not a reason" to "very important reason." Table 5.9 presents the percentage of drinkers who cited each reason as "very important" or "somewhat important." The data show that males were more likely to cite reasons as important for their drinking than were females, with the difference significant in five of the eight instances.

TABLE 5.9. Percent of Respondents Citing Very and Somewhat Important in Positive Reasons for Self Drinking by Gender

Very important reason	Male (N = 284)	Female (N = 290)	Total (N = 574)
1. I drink because there isn't anything else to do	12.7	4.8	8.7***
2. It is part of a good diet	5.6	3.1	4.4
3. I like the feeling of getting high or drunk	34.3	23.1	28.6**
4. Drinking helps me forget about my worries and problems.	20.1	16.2	18.1
5. Drinking gives me more confidence and makes me sure of myself	14.4	10.3	12.4
6. I drink when I feel tense or nervous	25.7	15.2	20.4**
7. I drink to be sociable	59.7	43.4	51.5***
8. I enjoy drinking	52.8	31.4	42.0***
Mean	2.25	1.47	$t = 5.38$***

* $p < .05$;   ** $p < .01$;   *** $p < .001$.

Pearson correlations between level of alcohol use and number of positive reasons for self-drinking indicates that the number of rationales for drinking is positively related to the amount of drinking. This relationship is similar for males (.33, $p < .001$) and females (.30, $p < .000$). Correlations between positive reasons for self-drinking and alcohol problems were stronger for males ($r = .45$, $p < .001$) than for females ($r = .33$, $p < .001$).

RATIONALES FOR CURTAILMENT OF DRINKING

From a list of 11 reasons, all respondents were asked to choose those that were important for their own abstinence or their "being careful about how much they drink." The responses ranged from "not a reason" to "very important reason." Table 5.10 presents the percentage of abstainers and drinkers who cited each reason as "very important." For each item, abstainers were more likely than drinkers to cite the reason as "very important." The differences between drinkers and abstainers were significant for all reasons.

When examining the differences between males and females separately for abstainers and drinkers (see Table 5.11), we find that for each item abstainers are still more likely to state that the reason was very important than were the drinkers. Only work concerns differentiated male and female abstainers, while for the drinkers five concerns are significantly different (with a higher percentage of concern in each case for females). The t-test difference between male and female means for number of reasons given was significant for drinkers only.

These rationales for the control of ones' drinking may be viewed as possibly predisposing respondents to curtail drinking. One hypothesis tested was whether the more rationales one has for curtailing drinking (or the more negative attitudes one has about drinking) is correlated

TABLE 5.10. Percent of Respondents Citing Very Important in Reasons for Abstaining
or Curtailing Drinking by Drinker

Very important reason	Male (N = 493)	Female (N = 574)	Total (N = 1067)
1. Drinking is bad for your health	90.5	73.3	81.3***
2. It costs too much when you need money for other things	71.5	61.8	66.3***
3. Drinking leads to losing control over your life	65.7	53.9	59.3***
4. It may interfere with your job or work	61.5	55.1	58.1*
5. Drinking can get you into trouble with the police or authorities	61.1	51.2	55.8**
6. Drinking can make you feel sick	64.6	42.7	52.9***
7. You are afraid of becoming an alcoholic	59.8	41.0	49.7***
8. Drinking can make you feel tired and depressed	55.0	37.9	45.8***
9. Drinking often makes you do things you are sorry for later	57.1	35.4	45.4***
10. It goes against your religion	59.1	27.2	41.9***
11. Your family or friends get upset when you drink	47.6	31.4	38.8***
Mean	6.90	5.10	$t = 8.16$***

* $p < .05$;   ** $p < .01$;   *** $p < .001$.

with a lower likelihood of extensive drinking. Our data indicate that among drinkers the greater the number of negative attitudes, the less extensive the drinking ($r = -.19$, $p < .001$). This was found to be true for both males ($r = -.16$, $p < .01$) and females ($r = -.19$, $p < .01$). Whether those who drink less develop socially protective rationales for doing so while living in a prodrinking Anglo culture or whether socially learned attitudes help curtail drinking cannot be deduced from these data.

When correlating the number of reasons for curtailing drinking with the number of positive reasons for self-drinking we find the relationship is in the expected direction; that is, as the number of reasons to drink

TABLE 5.11. Percent of Respondents Citing Very Important in Reasons for Abstaining or Curtailing Drinking by Gender and Drinkers

Very important reason	Abstainers		Drinkers	
	Male (N = 148)	Female (N = 345)	Male (N = 284)	Female (N = 290)
1. Drinking is bad for your health	88.5	91.3	69.4	77.2*
2. It costs too much when you need money for other things	69.6	72.4	54.6	69.0***
3. Drinking leads to losing control over your life	71.6	63.1	50.7	57.1
4. It may interfere with your job or work	69.7	58.0**	56.6	53.7
5. Drinking can get you into trouble with the police or authorities	66.2	58.9	48.9	53.4
6. Drinking can make you feel sick	64.6	64.6	38.0	47.2*
7. You are afraid of becoming an alcoholic	64.2	57.8	34.6	47.2**
8. Drinking can make you feel tired and depressed.	57.4	53.9	32.0	43.8**
9. Drinking often makes you do things you are sorry for later	60.8	55.5	32.4	38.3
10. It goes against your religion	58.1	59.5	23.9	30.3
11. Your family or friends get upset when you drink	50.3	46.1	32.9	30.0
Mean	7.19	6.77^a	4.73	5.46b

* $p < .05$;   ** $p < .01$;   *** $p < .001$.
^{a} ($t = 1.13$, df = 491, $p > .05$) ^{b} ($t = -2.57$, d f= 572, $p < .01$).

increases, the number of positive rationales for drinking decreases ($r = .23, p < .001$). This was true for both males ($r = -.19, p < .001$) and females ($r = -.25, p < .001$) although somewhat stronger for females.

What is the relationship between these negative attitudes, about drinking (presented in Table 5.11) and the drinking problems of male and female drinkers? It would be useful for development of action and prevention intervention models if we could find evidence that as negative attitudes about drinking increase, less drinking problems appear in the population, but this is not what the data show. We found no significant differences in the number of negative attitudes regarding drinking and the number of drinking problems for women ($r = .09$, $p > .05$). However, differences were found among men ($r = .23$, $p < .001$) but not in the expected direction. That is, men with more negative views regarding alcohol had a higher number of problems. Thus, the expected negative relationship between curtailment rationales and alcohol problems did not occur for either males or females. Even if one argues that a higher degree of problems may have produced the more negative views, we believe that the importance of these findings should not be minimized.

All too often, preventive education programs for alcohol and other drugs have stressed the negative consequences of substance use in the guise of "educating" young persons to the end of reducing use and consequent problems. Preventive education programs based on negative emphases long have been criticized and even longer have been carried out. They have ranged from the "Mickey Mouse" scare cartoons (programs to prevent sexually transmitted diseases through abstinence presented to American service personnel in World War II and the Korean War) to the "Partnership for Drug Free America" commercials showing substance users "freaking out." Certainly, in the area of substance abuse during the last few decades, there has been much fluctuation for all substance use but little overall diminution of use by youth. The substance of choice may vary from year to year and illicit substances may go down while alcohol use goes up, but no apparent and socially significant reduction has been found when both are considered. Few persons other than politicians would argue that "scare" prevention programs have had much if any impact on the totality of substance abuse by youth. In our observations and opinion, the history of preventive education indicates that when socially and politically defined negative consequences contradict the personal experiences and observations of youths and adults, messages are likely to be rejected. It is folly to believe that information to the young on the dangers of marijuana, alcohol, psychedelics, opiates, sedatives, and stimulants can achieve the reduction in substance use that this society would like to achieve. Even with the overpowering images, information, and data of the real physical dangers of cigarette smoking, the appeal to young persons to stop smoking has had only small and slow positive results. Lacking the strength of such information, substance abuse prevention programs are more often than not taken with the proverbial "grain of salt" or worse, treated as downright lies of the "establishment." While answers to the problems of alcohol and substance abuse may not be readily at hand, a negative and punitive approach has done little but impede attempts at a search for rational, effective, and humane solutions.

SITUATIONAL DRINKING RESTRAINTS

Respondents were asked questions regarding how much alcohol men and women should "feel free to drink" in certain situations (at parties, at bars, with family members, etc.) and at different ages (about 16, 21, 30, 40, and 60 years of age). The responses available were "no drinking," "1–2 drinks," "high but not drunk," and "sometimes drunk." These questions can be viewed as reflecting the constraints the respondents see existing in the culture regarding acceptable levels of drinking (see Table 5.12).

The items for which there was the most sentiment for abstinence were items 1–4. These four are directly related to personal responsibility in which drunkenness might jeopardize family, job, or cause injury. For

TABLE 5.12. Percent of Respondents Ranking Permissibility of Drinking in
Various Situations (Excluding Abstainers)
(*N* = 573)

How much drinking is all right...	No drinking	1 or 2 drinks	Enough to feel effects	Getting drunk is sometimes alright
1. When going to drive a car	93.4	6.5	0.2	0.0
2. During working hours, not just at lunch.	91.3	8.0	0.5	0.2
3. As a parent spending time with small children	76.8	21.4	1.7	0.0
4. For a couple of co-workers out to lunch.	75.8	23.0	1.2	0.0
5. When getting together with friends after work, before going home	48.9	41.9	8.2	1.0
6. When getting together with people at sports events or recreation	28.5	57.4	13.3	0.7
7. For a women out at a bar with friends	23.0	54.8	20.8	1.4
8. For a group of women that are out together	17.1	58.9	22.8	1.2
9. For a wife having dinner out with her husband	15.2	79.8	5.1	0.0
10. For a husband having dinner out with his wife	13.4	81.3	5.1	0.2
11. When with friends at home	11.5	64.6	22.0	1.9
12. At a party at someone else's home	5.9	65.9	26.1	2.1
13. For a man out at a bar with friends	5.8	43.6	43.6	4.0
14. For a group of men that are out together	4.5	45.5	46.7	3.3

these responsibility items (1–4), there are no significant differences
between men and women (data not shown). The largest support for

drinking to get high or even drunk is shown for those activities in which women are out with "the girls" and men are together with "the boys" (these are items 7, 8, 13, and 14, with males more than twice as likely to have permission to get high or drunk: 47.6% and 50.0% vs. 22.2% and 24.0%). This is followed by social gatherings at their own or someone else's home (items 11 and 12). It is interesting to note that less leeway is granted to wives having dinner with their husbands or vice versa (a socially structured situation in which drunkenness would be shameful) than either sex is permitted when they are out in more tolerant situations with their own gender (cf. item 9 with 7 and 8 for women and item 10 with 13 and 14 for men).

Do Puerto Rican men and women differ in their interpretation of the degree of permission allowed to each when they are out with their friends or at a bar (see Table 5.13)? As shown in Table 5.13, the differences in permissiveness between males and females regarding the level of drinking by men and women at bars and drinking when out with other members of the same sex is small. Both sexes agree that men at bars or out with other men have more permission to drink to get high or drunk than women in the same circumstances, although males are slightly more tolerant of men getting drunk when out than females are. It is interesting to note that males are also slightly more tolerant of women getting high or drunk than the females are.

Respondents also were asked to rank the limits on varying degrees of drinking for men and women at different ages. The results are consistent with the previous findings that greater tolerance is directed toward male drinking at different ages than female drinking (see Table 5.14). Greatest tolerances for both sexes are seen for the adult ages of 30s and 40s but there appears to be little tolerance for elderly people drinking. We know of no special cultural norm that places restriction on older persons drinking outside of the controls on female drinking in

TABLE 5.13. Percent of Males and Females Approving Varying Drinking Levels for Men and Women in Different Situations

	Males (N=283)				Females (N=290)			
	No drinks	1-2 drinks	Feel effects	Get drunk	No drinks	1-2 drinks	Feel effects	Get drunk
7. For a woman at bar	25.1	49.8	23.3	1.8	21.0	59.7	18.3	1.0
8. Women out together	19.7	53.9	25.0	1.4	14.5	63.8	20.7	1.0
13. For a man at bar	3.9	40.7	49.6	5.7	7.6	46.4	43.6	2.4
14. For men out together	2.8	44.0	48.9	4.2	6.2	46.9	44.5	2.4

general. Why this would extend to elderly male drinking cannot be ascertained from the data. One speculation that has arisen in the United States in recent years concerns the negative attitudes of middle-aged persons about the legitimacy of their widowed parents maintaining an active sex life. The analysis given is that it is subconscious "payback" time for earlier parental control over their children's sexual activities. It is not a stretch to imagine alcohol attitudes toward the elderly in the same vein. This is supported by the finding that there is greater tolerance for drinking for both men and women "about 60 years old" among those aged 55+ (78.5% for older men, 49.5% for older women) than among those under age 55 (49.7% for older men, 36.1% for older women).

TABLE 5.14. Percent of Respondents Ranking Limits on Drinking for Men and Women of Different Ages (Excluding Abstainers)

What is the most that each of these kinds of people should drink at one time?	No drinking	1 or 2 drinks	Enough to feel effects	Getting drunk is sometimes alright
1. A boy about 16 years old	91.3	8.2	.5	.0
2. A young man about 21 years old	17.2	70.6	11.0	1.2
3. A man about 30 years old	4.2	51.7	41.9	2.3
4. A man about 40 years old	7.4	47.6	41.0	4.0
5. A man about 60 years old	45.6	43.0	8.9	2.4
6. A girl about 16 years old	93.6	6.1	.2	.2
7. A young woman about 21 years old	26.5	66.0	7.0	.5
8. A woman about 30 years old	9.6	67.7	21.8	.9
9. A woman about 40 years old	18.6	59.8	20.0	1.6
10. A woman about 60 years old	62.0	31.6	5.4	1.0

ALCOHOLISM AND DRUNKS

Much of the outreach efforts to bring Hispanic alcoholics into treatment have derived from Anglo models in the literature, in which the notion of alcoholism as a disease has been stressed. This reflects the movement within the field of alcoholism treatment and research during the second half of the 20th century in which a medical model of addiction replaced the older views of the drunk as a weak willed and sometimes immoral individual (Heather & Robinson, 1981; Trice & Roman, 1970, 1978).

To ascertain current Puerto Rican attitudes and perceptions in this area, respondents were asked whether they agreed or disagreed with a number of statements and beliefs regarding alcoholics and drunks. The percent of drinkers and abstainers agreeing with each statement is presented in Table 5.15.

In general, abstainers had a more severe and punitive view of alcoholism and drunkenness than drinkers did. That is, abstainers were more likely to see all individuals who drink as vulnerable to becoming alcoholics, to view abstinence as required for recovery from alcoholism, and more likely to view the alcoholic as morally weak. Abstainers were not as likely to view drunkenness as "an innocent way of having fun" or as doing people some good. They also were more likely to be punitive and rejecting of "drunks" (see Table 5.15), but the largest gap between drinkers and abstainers is reflected in the presentation of self and family in the community (item 10).

How did the gender of the respondent impact the views regarding alcoholism and drunkenness? Table 5.16 presents responses the alcoholism and drunkenness statements for abstainers and drinkers according to gender.

TABLE 5.15. Percent of Drinkers and Abstainers Agreeing with Statements on
Alcoholism and Drunkenness

Very important reason	Male (N = 493)	Female (N = 574)	Total (N = 1067)
Alcoholism			
1. Alcoholism is an illness	94.1	93.0	93.5
2. Anyone who drinks can become an alcoholic	88.4	74.1	80.7***
3. Most alcoholics drink because they want to	54.3	54.0	54.1
4. To recover, alcoholics will have to quit drinking forever.	93.5	85.0	85.0***
5. Many alcoholics taper off and get their drinking under control again	62.5	57.0	59.5
6. The alcoholic is a morally weak individual	92.3	84.8	88.3***
Drunkenness			
7. Getting drunk is just an innocent way of having fun	23.4	31.6	27.8**
8. A man who is always drunk should be punished	44.2	35.8	39.7**
9. It does some people good to get drunk once in a while	6.5	19.9	13.7***
10. I would feel ashamed if anyone in my family got drunk	89.4	68.1	77.9***
11. A drunk person is a disgusting sight	83.0	69.5	75.8***
12. People who get drunk can be very amusing	67.9	67.4	67.6
13. Someone who is drunk and punches someone else should get the same punishment he'd get if he were sober	60.4	60.2	60.3

$*p < .05;$ $**p < .01;$ $***p < .001.$

TABLE 5.16. Percent of Abstainers and Drinkers Stating They Agree with Statements on Alcoholism and Drunkenness by Gender

	Abstainer		Drinker	
Statement	Male (N = 147)	Female (N = 344)	Male (N = 284)	Female (N = 289)
Alcoholism				
1. Alcoholism is an illness	92.5	94.8	92.2	93.8
2. Anyone who drinks can become an alcoholic	82.3	91.0**	73.1	75.1
3. Most alcoholics drink because they want to	50.3	56.0	51.2	56.6
4. To recover, alcoholics will have to quit drinking forever	91.8	94.2	80.6	89.3**
5. Many alcoholics taper off and get their drinking under control again	55.8	65.4*	54.8	59.2
6. The alcoholic is a morally weak individual	87.8	94.2*	80.6	88.9*
Drunkenness				
7. Getting drunk is just an innocent way of having fun	25.0	22.7	34.9	28.4
8. A man who is always drunk should be punished	36.1	47.7*	35.3	36.3
9. It does some people good to get drunk once in a while	10.8	4.7*	27.1	12.8**
10. I would feel ashamed if anyone in my family got drunk	85.0	91.3*	59.9	76.3**
11. A drunk person is a disgusting sight	80.3	84.2	66.1	72.9
12. People who get drunk can be very amusing	67.8	67.9	71.6	63.3*
13. Someone who is drunk and punches someone else should get the same punishment he'd get if he were sober	58.8	61.2	63.7	56.7

*p < .05;   **p < .01;   ***p < .001.

Men appear to be more accepting of the behavior and consequences of drunkenness than were women. Males were more likely than females to view drunks as amusing and to see drunkenness as a good thing once in a while. Males also were significantly less likely to consider punishment for a man that is always drunk, be ashamed of a drunken family member, and find drunken individuals a "disgusting sight." On the other hand, women were more sensitive to the public image and reaction to drunkenness.

The ambivalence regarding the nature of addiction, in this case alcoholism, in American society is captured by the high percentage of individuals who stated that alcoholism is an illness and the high percentage of individuals stating that the alcoholic is morally weak. Analysis of these responses revealed that 84% of the respondents (82.2% of abstainers and 79.3% of drinkers) held both views. In fact, there are five paired contradictions in the list: 1–6, 4–5, 7–8, 9–10, and 11–12. It is reasonable to speculate that these contradictions may be a function of the differences in images of drinking between an older more traditional view of drinking and drinkers held on "the Island" and the confused state of Anglo mores that present no monolithic view of drinking norms. In order to test this, drinkers were ranked by the number of contradictory positions held by adding the agreements for each pair. This then was correlated with their degree of acculturation and traditionalism.

We found that as the level of acculturation increased the number of contradictory statements regarding alcoholism and drunkenness decreased for both males and females ($r = -.28$, $p < .001$ and $r = -.21$, $p < .001$, respectively). On the other hand, we found that as the level of traditionalism increased so did the number of contradictory images ($r = .24$, $p < .001$ for males and $r = .17$, $p < .001$ for females). This may suggest that the images and definitions of alcoholism and drunkenness in the Hispanic (Puerto Rican) culture differs from that of Anglos creating confusion and contradictory images for persons who are at the early stages of acculturation or who still adhere to the traditional Island norms.

THE SEARCH FOR HELP

Researchers have found reluctance among many Hispanics to seek treatment for substance abuse and other compulsive behavior problems. Among the reasons suggested for this unwillingness are shame of exposure, gender norms (inhibiting males from acknowledging they have a problem and impeding females from seeking help due to fear of consequences within the family and community), distrust of governmental agencies or other official services, lack of understanding about where to go for treatment, and confusion about different treatment options (Arredondo, Weddige, Justice, & Fitz, 1987; Canino, Anthony, Freeman, Shrout, & Rubio-Stipec, 1993; Cuadrado, 1999; Gloria & Peregoy, 1996; Panitz et al., 1983).

All drinkers were asked several questions about their attitudes concerning seeking treatment for drinking problems. Less than one third (29.2%) of the drinkers stated that they would be ashamed to tell someone about their own drinking problem. Few respondents (9.2%) reported that they did not know where to get help for a drinking problem and almost all (98.4%) viewed alcohol problems as likely to be progressive and requiring help. There were no significant differences between males and females on these items.

Respondents also were asked whether they had ever talked about an alcohol problem of their own with anyone and if they had ever gone for help. Among those respondents who had stated in previous questions that they had at least one alcohol problem, we found that less than a fifth (18.7%) of the respondents had discussed their problem with someone, with no significant differences between men and women. Only 10.0% of the respondents with at least one problem had gone for help, with males about twice as likely to go as females (11.7% vs. 5.6%), but the difference was not statistically significant due to the small number of cases.

One likely explanation for men being more willing to go for help is that among the group of respondents who had at least one problem, men on average had a significantly higher number of problems than women (8.02 vs. 4.75, $t = 3.13$, df $= 251$, $p < .01$). In addition, males with problems were over four times as likely to report employment problems than females (18.9% vs. 4.2%, $p < .01$), almost twice as likely to have problems with the family (55.8% vs. 30.6%, $p < .001$), and more likely to report antisocial behavior problems than females (45.9% vs. 31.0%). These types of problems expose the drinker to others (i.e., employers, family members, and police) who are more likely to exert pressure on the person to seek treatment. The employment variable needs some clarification. To insure that the difference between men and women regarding employment problems was not due to being unemployed (which women are more likely to be), we redid the analysis only among individuals with at least one problem who were currently employed. We found that 17.7% of the males and none of the females had employment problems ($N = 146$, $p < .05$).

Of the 47 respondents who talked with someone about their own alcohol problems, the largest group (72.4%) spoke to their friends, followed by spouse (61.7%), doctor (55.3%) and relatives other than spouse (51.1%). Religious ministers were among the least mentioned (17.0%). As for the 25 persons who actually sought help, they turned to Alcoholics Anonymous (65.2%), general hospitals (64.7%), other alcohol programs (44.0%), and private physicians (44.0%).

Were the remaining respondents with drinking problems who did not talk with someone or go for help more likely to be those who were ashamed, did not know where to go for help or who did not believe that alcohol problems were progressive? Apparently not. Among those 201 respondents who did not talk with anyone about their drinking problem or go for help, less than a third (30.3%) reported that they would be

ashamed of telling anyone, almost 90% knew where to get help, and
96.5% viewed alcohol problems as progressive. There were no statistical
differences between men and women.

Thus, ignorance of resources, greater shame, or belief in a
nonprogressive view of alcohol problems appears not to explain the lack
of seeking treatment. One difficulty of interpretation of data such as the
self-reporting data used in this study lies in the discrepancy between the
"subjective meaning" of responses as they are relevant to the lifestyle
and culture of respondents and the more objective and scientific criteria
imposed on that data by the researcher. Respondents had been asked in
this study if they ever had "some experiences many people have
reported in connection with drinking." It is the response to these items
(presented in Table 4.9) that has been classified as "problems" in keeping
with the traditional model of alcoholism used in these analyses. This
"medical model" follows the conventional medical beliefs that
alcoholism is a progressive disease manifested in part by the problems
developed in connection with drinking. Whether an individual is an
alcoholic or not is not the focus of this study, since alcohol addiction has
different theoretical explanations with many proponents of dissimilar
and at times contradictory approaches to etiology and treatment
(Fingarette, 1989; Heather & Robinson, 1981; Jellinek, 1960; Kishline,
1994; Lewis, Dana, & Blevins, 1988; Peele, 1989; Rudy, 1986; Trimpey,
1989). All that can be said safely at this point is that these are the
consequences that may accrue from drinking for some respondents
independent of whether or not there is any physical or psychological
dependence. The problem raised by this designation of the 35 situations
or events as problematic is that these reflect the opinions and biases of
most alcoholism practitioners and researchers but not necessarily the
respondents. Thus, even though we may operationalize the degree of
problem drinking with the aid of the Index of Alcohol Problems, in some
or even many cases the respondents may not have shared our views that
these were "problems." Therefore, the low percentage of individuals

seeking treatment may reflect a sharp difference in the cultural definitions of what are acceptable and what are problematic behaviors before, during, and as a consequence of alcohol consumption.

The issue of definition of problematic behavior is one that is central to those in the field who are interested in prevention and outreach work among Hispanics, for it makes the task more complicated. Prevention and outreach efforts need not only concentrate on providing information on how to get help, but often must define the problem. This definition, though, must take into account the culture and definition of the situation of the group being addressed. An example from the experiences of the authors in a different area of compulsive disorders: problem or compulsive gambling. Brochures, advertisements, billboards, and so forth, designed to inform the Hispanic communities as to the existence of problem gambling and that help is available, often are a literal Spanish translation of the English sources, where the term "gambling addiction" may be used. Calling what may be perceived by Hispanics as recreational gambling behavior an addiction is likely to be a turnoff within the Puerto Rican community already worried by clear and unequivocal heroin addiction. (Similarly, calling heavy drinking by men and the use of marijuana an addiction likely may not be taken seriously in the Puerto Rican community or many other Latin American groups.) Many Puerto Ricans tend to view gambling, even "excessive" gambling, especially horse races, cockfights, lottery, *la bolita*, and dominoes as innocent fun and recreation. Labeling or demonizing these behaviors as sinister and an addiction may be counterproductive. Similarly, the designations of customary alcohol behaviors as alcohol problems should be approached cautiously when researching Hispanic and all populations.

IMPACT OF ACCULTURATION AND TRADITIONALISM

What have been the substance use, misuse, and abuse consequences for Puerto Ricans of becoming "Anglocized" or more like their English speaking counterparts on the mainland? Is substance misuse and the abuse problems arising from this a result of the striving to be like "everyone else" and integrating into the larger Anglo community? Which parts of this transition process are most related to substance misuse and abuse? Is the movement toward substance misuse and abuse merely a matter of time spent on the mainland or differences in education and class that result in the stresses of acculturation? Are the substance abuse problems of Puerto Ricans on the mainland more a product of the stresses resulting from their striving to "fit in" or during this process have they lost their commitment to certain traditional values that had served to protect them on "the Island?"

ACCULTURATION, TRADITIONALISM, AND OUTCOMES

As we stated earlier, the main focus of this volume is to explore whether the degree of acculturation alone, or the degree of loss of traditional values alone, or a high degree of acculturation in combination with the loss of traditional values provides the best explanation for drinking and drug use behaviors and their consequences among Puerto Ricans. In this chapter we will examine the impact of acculturation and traditionalism separately in the areas of: (1) alcohol use: abstention and level; (2) extent of drinking in different settings: number of places and extent; (3) number of drinking problems and areas of problems; and (4) drug use. The combined effects of acculturation and traditionalism will be examined in the next chapter.

ALCOHOL USE: ABSTENTION AND LEVEL

Over the years, many researchers have found that when it comes to choosing to drink, the impact of acculturation is far greater for women than it is for men (Alcocer, 1982; Black & Markides, 1993; Caetano, 1984a,b, 1986, 1987a; Caetano & Medina Mora, 1988; Canino, 1994; Graves, 1967; Lovato, Litrownik, Elder, & Nunez-Liriano, 1994; Madsen, 1964; Marin & Posner, 1995; Page et al., 1985). Our findings, presented in Table 6.1, confirm this. Although the degree of acculturation is found to be significantly related to the choice of alcohol use reported by both men and women (as the level of acculturation increased, so did the likelihood of being a drinker), the impact of acculturation on this relationship is over twice as strong for women as for men ($r = .26$ versus $r = .12$).

Traditionalism levels also were found to be related to the likelihood of being a drinker: the higher the level of traditionalism the lower the likelihood of being a drinker. However, the relationship is significant only for women. Although Puerto Rican tradition has been said to "encourage" male drinking, males who are more traditional are not significantly more likely to be drinkers.

TABLE 6.1. Percent of Abstainers by Degree of Acculturation and Loss of Traditional Family Role Attitudes (Traditionalism A) by Gender[a]

	Male[b]				Female[b]			
	Low	Med	High	Total	Low	Med	High	Total
Acculturation								
Abstainers	46.3	31.3	29.3	34.3	69.4	46.3	42.3	54.3
Drinkers	53.7	68.7	70.7	65.7	30.6	53.7	57.7	45.7
	$N = 432, r = .12, p < .01$				$N = 635, r = .26, p < .001$			
Traditionalism A								
Abstainers	26.4	36.2	37.2	34.3	52.0	49.5	61.7	54.3
Drinkers	73.6	63.8	62.8	65.7	48.0	50.5	38.3	45.7
	$N = 432, r = -.06, p > .05$				$N = 635, r = -.09, p < .05$			

[a] Acculturation and traditionalism A grouped into discrete categories for the purpose of presentation. Correlations were obtained from unrecoded versions of the variables.
[b] Numbers are percents.

When we examine only those respondents who are drinkers, we find that the relationships between acculturation or traditionalism and level of drinking are not significant for either males or females. For women, however, having a more traditional outlook indicates a strong tendency toward having a braking effect on the degree of drinking: 49.3% of high traditionalism women were scored as low on alcohol use compared to 30.0% of low traditionalism women. For males, the percentages were 24.4% for high traditionals and 17.9% for low traditionals.

DRINKING IN DIFFERENT SETTINGS: NUMBER OF PLACES AND EXTENT

Opportunities for drinking are somewhat different for Puerto Rican men and women on "the Island" compared with mainland United States. This is mainly due to the relatively greater acceptance of male drinking in most circumstances in Puerto Rico and the very limited acceptance of any public drinking for traditional Puerto Rican women compared to the acceptability of many public drinking situations for both men and women in mainland United States. In order to learn whether greater public acceptance resulted in greater public participation in drinking for women, we examined the number of different places (restaurants, clubs, bars, parties, and parks or street) at which nonabstaining respondents may drink. Many of these places are public and would result in women being observed by others in her community. We found that higher levels of acculturation were significantly related to drinking at a greater number of places among the males ($r = .16, p < .01$) but not among the females ($r = .05, p > .05$) (see Table 6.2). Males who scored "high" on the Acculturation Index were more likely to also score "high" on the Different Settings index. This was also true of women but the unrecoded correlations were found not to be significant.

Higher traditionalism levels were negatively related to the number of places at which women drinkers tended to drank ($r = -.22, p < .001$). Traditionalism appears to curb the number of places women are willing to be seen as drinkers. Traditionalism was not significantly related with the number of drinking places among men. Among male drinkers, those with low levels of traditionalism were more likely to cite a higher number of drinking places than those with high levels of traditionalism but the unrecoded correlations were not found to be significant ($r = -.08, p > .05$) (see Table 6.2).

An interesting finding is the effect of traditionalism on the possibility of developing drinking problems. Researchers have suggested that there may be a likelihood of the development of problem drinking among persons who drink in a new cultural setting if they come from cultures which prohibit drinking (Lafferty, Holden, & Klein, 1980; Larsen & Abu-Laban, 1968; Pittman, 1967; Skolnick, 1958; Ullman, 1958). In part, this may be due to the fact that these drinkers have not been "socialized" into the new normative drinking patterns, i.e., they have not learned the "hows" of limit setting based on the new drinking group's norms in

Table 6.2. Extent of Drinking in Different Settings by Degree of
Acculturation and Traditional Family Role Attitudes (Traditionalism A) by
Gender[a]

	Male[b]				Female[b]			
	Low	Med	High	Total	Low	Med	High	Total
Extent of drinking in different settings				Acculturation				
Low (score 9–12)	45.1	32.4	26.4	32.3	58.7	41.1	39.8	45.2
Med. (score 13–16)	17.6	28.4	22.7	24.0	27.0	34.6	34.6	32.6
High (score 17–36)	37.3	38.2	50.9	43.7	14.3	24.3	25.6	22.2
	$N = 263, r = .16, p < .01$				$N = 248, r = .05, p > .05$			
				Traditionalism A				
Low (score 9–12)	19.7	34.6	39.7	32.3	36.4	49.4	56.3	45.2
Med. (score 13–16)	22.4	18.5	29.2	24.0	37.2	30.1	27.3	32.6
High (score 17–36)	57.9	46.9	31.1	43.7	26.4	20.5	16.4	22.2
	$N = 263, r = -.08, p > .05$				$N = 248, r = -.22, p < .001$			

[a] Acculturation and traditionalism A grouped into discrete categories for the purpose
of presentation. Correlations were obtained from unrecoded versions of the variables.
[b] Numbers are percents.

combination with the uncertain newly found physiological responses to
the alcohol itself. One might say that their "set" and "setting" are
inappropriate to deal with the new situation in which they now find
themselves.

In this study, we have had an opportunity to see the effect of this on traditional Puerto Rican women. They have been socialized within a set of proscriptive norms controlling all aspects of drinking, similar to abstinence norms described by Pittman (1967). During the process of acculturation these women move into an Anglo culture that has been classified by Pittman (1967) as ambivalent in its norms regarding drinking and that does not provide the needed guidelines for appropriate drinking with respect to time, frequency, amount, and setting. Hence, there are no consistent regulating norms within the Anglo community held up as a model for female drinkers. As suggested by the above researchers, traditional values, which may have prevented or curtailed the drinking among women, may not have any effect on preventing or curtailing the occurrence of problems once they begin to drink. Our data do not support this conclusion for Puerto Rican women. In Table 6.3, we see that there are no significant differences between traditionalism and drinking problems for the more highly traditional women.

The strongest relationship between traditionalism and any of the drinking outcome variables for women was found with extent of drinking in different settings ($r = -.22, p < .001$). That is, the higher the level of traditionalism, the less likely women were to drink in different settings. This may be expected for women, since the drinking norms that the Puerto Rican culture imposes on women do not prevent them from drinking in a prescribed setting, but drinking in other nonnormative settings will expose her to the scrutiny of the community. Drinking in different public settings would be considered an obvious breach of those behaviors that a traditional woman would not likely engage in even if she is a drinker(Aguirre-Molina, 1991). However, a ranking of low on drinking in different settings does not necessarily mean the avoidance of problematic drinking. Despite significant correlations between extent of drinking in different setting and alcohol problems for both males and females ($r = .17, p < .01$ for males and $r = .20, p < .01$ for women), analysis of the relationship between drinking problems and extent of drinking in different settings indicates that 44.6% of men and 16.8% of women who were low in extent of drinking had at least one alcohol problem.

Fernandez-Pol et al. (1986) found that Puerto Rican women who were problem drinkers tended to drink alone in the privacy of their homes (a drinking behavior that cannot come under community scrutiny, and thus may not be perceived as a violation of traditional norms). This practice may be a red flag for possible indications of more clearly defined problems that arise regarding drinking. This is supported by our finding that women who drank at home ("spending a quiet evening at home") were twice as likely as those who did not drink at home to have an alcohol problem [16.4% versus 32.1%, $\chi^2(1, N = 283) =$ 9.43, $p < .01$]. A Puerto Rican woman who drinks alone away from the scrutiny of the community also will likely be a woman that will not seek help or treatment if the need were to arise because of the harsh stigma attached to being a drunk or *borrachona*.

DRINKING PROBLEMS

There are many kinds of problems that may result from drinking irrespective of the amount and frequency of consumption. One drinker may consume little alcohol but may seem to be much more affected by the drinking than another who consumes a great deal but is considered able to "hold his liquor." As discussed in Chapter 5, respondents were asked if they had ever had each of 35 different experiences that they could attribute to their drinking. These experiences have been designated for the purposes of this volume as "alcohol problems." (See discussion of this issue at end of Chapter 5.)

Among male drinkers, both the level of acculturation and the degree of traditionalism were found to be significantly related to the number of drinking problems. Males scored as "low" on the Acculturation Index were more likely to have at least one drinking problem than men with higher levels of acculturation (67.1% vs. 48.4%; $r = -.26$, $p < .001$), while males with higher levels of traditionalism were more likely to have at least one problem (43% vs. 56.3%; $r = .16$, $p < .01$) (see Table 6.3). As males become more acculturated and as they become less traditional, they lessen their likelihood of problematic drinking. For women the findings are quite different from those among men, i.e., acculturation and traditionalism are not significantly correlated with drinking problems.

What may account for more acculturated male drinkers being less likely to have alcohol problems than less acculturated? Probably the same factors that account for the more traditional men being more likely to have alcohol problems than less traditional male drinkers. The more acculturated male is in a position to better learn the non-Puerto Rican community responses—police, employers, neighbors, Anglo friends—to drunkenness and inappropriate drinking than his counterpart who is less exposed to them. Similarly, the more traditional male may still be drinking with the attitudes carried over from the more permissive toleration of excessive male drinking in Puerto Rico. Inappropriate drinking and drunkenness would jeopardize the more acculturated male's standing in the Anglo community in which he is operating and relating.

How do acculturation and traditionalism relate to each individual problem? Table 6.4 presents the correlations between the separate problems cited by respondents due to drinking (grouped according to area) and acculturation and traditionalism.

Table 6.3. Number of Problems Due to Drinking by Degree of Acculturation and Traditional Family Role Attitudes (Traditionalism A) by Gender[a]

	Male[b]				Female[b]			
	Low	Med	High	Total	Low	Med	High	Total
Number of problems			Acculturation					
None	32.9	49.5	51.6	46.6	82.4	75.4	71.2	75.8
Low (1)	7.9	11.5	17.4	13.0	6.3	8.2	13.4	9.4
Med. (2–6)	25.0	15.3	18.9	18.9	3.8	12.3	7.2	8.4
High (7+)	34.2	23.7	12.1	21.5	7.5	4.1	8.2	6.4

$N = 339, r = .-26, p < .001$ $\qquad$ $N = 299, r = .02, p > .05$

			Traditionalism A					
None	57.0	42.1	43.7	46.6	74.0	77.7	76.9	75.8
Low (1)	11.6	16.7	11.3	13.0	7.9	10.6	10.3	9.4
Med. (2–6)	15.1	16.7	22.5	18.9	9.4	8.5	6.4	8.4
High (7+)	16.3	24.5	22.5	21.5	8.7	3.2	6.4	6.4

$N = 339, r = .16, p < .01$ $\qquad$ $N = 299, r = -.06, p > .05$

[a] Acculturation and traditionalism A grouped into discrete categories for the purpose of presentation. Correlations were obtained from unrecoded versions of the variables.
[b] Numbers are percents.

TABLE 6.4. Correlations Between Each Problem Cited, Acculturation, and
Traditionalism A for Males and Females

Problems[a]	Acculturation		Traditionalism A	
	Male	Female	Male	Female
Family & social (at least 1 problem)	(N = 339)	(N = 299)	(N = 339)	(N = 299)
Drinking interfered with spare time activities or hobbies	-.16**	-.05	.05	.02
Spouse or mate angry about my drinking	-.15**	.11	.09	-.10
Spouse or mate threatened to leave because of my drinking	-.21***	.03	.08	-.10
Family and friends pressure to cut down on drinking	-.09	.05	.05	-.05
Employment (at least 1 problem)	(N = 338)	(N = 297)	(N = 338)	(N = 297)
Lost job or nearly lost job because of drinking	-.11*	.00	.11*	.05
Fellow workers suggested to curtail my drinking	-.15**	Insuff.	.10	Insuff.
Drinking hurt promotions, raises or better job	-.09	.08	.05	.05
Health (At least 1 problem)	(N=339)	(N=299)	(N=339)	(N=299)
Skipped meals while drinking	-.20***	.04	.09	-.04
Hands shook on morning after drinking	-.20***	-.04	.17**	-.03
Night time sweats due to drinking	-.16**	.05	.12*	-.03
Drinking related illness prevented normal work for week or more	-.23***	-.05	.12*	-.11
Believed drinking was seriously affecting health	-.23***	.03	.14**	-.12*
Physician suggested cut down on drinking	-.25***	.01	.11*	-.10
Fits or seizures after cessation or cutting down of drinking	-.14**	-.02	.12*	-.00
DTs (hallucinations and fever) after cessation of drinking	-.16**	-.05	.16**	.01

Seen or heard things not there after cutting down on drinking	-.16**	-.03	.10	-.05
Loss of control over drinking (At least 1 problem)	(N=339)	(N=299)	(N=339)	(N=299)
Often drink first thing after waking up	-.23***	-.03	.17**	-.03
Taken strong drink in morning to overcome hangover	-.24***	-.03	.12*	.00
Blackout of previous nights drinking	-.22***	.07	.07	-.03
Need more alcohol for same effects	-.19***	.04	.16**	.02
Needed a drink so bad I couldn't think of anything else	-.22***	.02	.17**	.01
Stayed intoxicated for several days at a time	-.18**	-.02	.15**	-.03
Once began drinking, continued until intoxicated	-.17**	.01	.15**	-.02
Continued drinking after promising self not to	-.16**	-.08	.09	-.01
Try to cut down but was unable to do so	-.17**	-.04	.03	-.03
Afraid I was an alcoholic	-.10	.14*	.09	-.10
Drinking 5 or more drinks at a sitting at least once a week	-.24***	-.05	.13*	-.06
Felt drinking was not under my control	-.23***	-.02	.10	-.07
Antisocial behavior (At least 1 problem)	(N=339)	(N=298)	(N=339)	(N=298)
Heated arguments while drinking	-.15**	.04	.10	-.07
Fights while drinking	-.17**	.07	.13*	-.05
Police officer questioned or warned me because of my drinking	-.14*	-.02	.06	.11*
Drinking led me to be hurt in car accident or elsewhere	-.11*	.04	.11*	.06
Drinking led to others hurt or property damage	-.07	.04	.00	.06

| Non-automobile trouble with law due to drink | -.08 | .02 | .05 | .07 |
| Arrested as for driving after drinking | -.04 | -.02 | -.01 | .01 |

* p < .05;   ** p < .01;   *** p < .001.
ᵃWording modified from questionnaire for brevity.

When we examine Table 6.4 we find that for males, all correlations are negative and most are significant, reflecting the importance of acculturation in the inhibition of problems for males. This is reinforced by the finding that almost twice as many of the correlations between problems and acculturation were statistically significant than the correlations between problems and traditionalism (29 vs. 17). The apparent influence of acculturation in the prevention of alcohol-related problems in all of the areas for males is striking. It suggests that additional research to sharply define the elements of acculturation that are most definitely related to the prevention of alcohol problems would be a worthwhile research undertaking that may have implications not only for Puerto Rican and other Hispanic males but perhaps even for other ethnic groups.

The highest correlation for males between the inhibition of a "drinking problem" and acculturation was "physician suggested cut down on drinking" ($r = -.25$). What could explain this negative correlation (and others as well)? One might be tempted to say the obvious, that those ranked "high" on acculturation drink less than those who scored low on acculturation. However, as discussed above, there is no correlation between acculturation and level of alcohol use. Another possibility is that the more highly acculturated males are physically healthier, and thus less likely to see doctors. Refusing to acknowledge the suggestions of doctors (or others) that they might have an alcohol problem (denial) because it is too threatening to the upward mobility of the more highly acculturated is another interesting possibility. Similarly, they might have learned more appropriate or ritual drinking, as suggested by Weil (1986), limiting their drinking to before dinner and during meals and ceremonial occasions only, thus cutting down on loss of control. One other explanation that lends itself to further research comes from one of the author's prior work and research with Jewish alcoholics, i.e., the possibility of misdiagnosis of problem drinking or alcoholism. This may occur with the Puerto Rican male because of the more middle class appearance that the "High Acculturated" male may present to an Anglo physician negating the stereotype of the lower-class "low acculturated" male that still retains the *macho* excessive drinking image associated with it. All these possible explanations could be productive research undertakings.

For the males in our sample, all Traditionalism A Index (attitudes) correlations were positive; that is, the higher the traditionalism score, the more likely males were to have cited one or more of these problems. The largest correlations with the Traditionalism A Index were "hands shook on morning after drinking," "often drink first thing after waking up," and "needed a drink so bad I couldn't think of anything else" (all with r = .17). These are all items of self-determinations and, with the possible exception of "lost job or nearly lost job because of drinking," none of the significant correlations were with items in which someone else in his social world had indicated that he might have an alcohol problem. This is consistent with the widely held notion that excessive alcohol consumption and consequences are usually accepted within the more traditional circles. This, of course, makes intervention much more difficult with a population not likely to recognize a problem among friends and compatriots.

Among women, the problems related to acculturation and traditionalism can be seen as based on nonspecific indicators of problematic drinking. The only correlation related to acculturation was

TABLE 6.5. Correlations between Grouped Problem Areas, Degree of
Acculturation, and Traditionalism A for Males and Females

Problem Areas	Acculturation		Traditionalism A	
	Male ($N = 339$)	Female ($N = 299$)	Male ($N = 339$)	Female ($N = 299$)
Family and social	-.18***	.06	.09	-.09
Employment	-.15**	.05	.11*	.07
Health	-.27***	.00	.17**	-.09
Loss of control	-.26***	.00	.15**	-.05
Antisocial behavior	-.18***	.05	.11*	.00

*$p < .05$;   **$p < .01$;   ***$p < .001$.

the generalized and vague "afraid I was an alcoholic" ($r = .14$) and for traditionalism the only positive correlation was "police officer questioned or warned me because of my drinking" ($r = .11$). This latter correlation may possibly indicate the great fear that traditional Puerto Rican women have of being seen as or labeled in the community as a *borrachona* (drunken woman).

In sum, acculturation seems to have a preventive role to play in inhibiting the development of male alcohol problems but the opposite is true for traditionalism where we find positive correlation with four of the five areas, i.e., the greater the traditionalism, the greater the likelihood of problems (see Table 6.5). For female drinkers, neither acculturation nor traditionalism is correlated with any problem area.

DRUG USE

Although research on Puerto Rican adult drug use is scarce, several research studies including this one (see discussion in Chapter 4) have shown that Puerto Rican men are more likely then Puerto Rican women to use drugs (Amaro et al., 1990; Austin & Gilbert, 1989; Booth et al., 1990). Do acculturation and traditionalism play a role in this? In Table 6.6 we find that the degree of acculturation is significantly related to the use of drugs during the 12 months prior to the interview for both men and women: the higher the level of acculturation, the more likely the use of illegal substances during that time. High acculturation males were nearly four times as likely as low acculturation males to use drugs, while high acculturation women were nearly 9 times as likely as low acculturated women to use drugs, and males at each level of acculturation were more likely than their female counterparts to use drugs.

The degree of traditionalism was found to be negatively related to the use of drugs during the 12 months prior to the interview for both men and women, i.e., the higher the level of traditionalism, the less likely men and women were to have used an illegal substance during that time period. Women with low levels of traditionalism were over twice as likely as women with high levels of traditionalism to have used drugs in

TABLE 6.6. Percent of Males and Females Using Illicit Drug in Past 12 Months by Degree of Acculturation and Traditionalism A[a]

	Male[b]				Female[b]			
	Low	Med	High	Total	Low	Med	High	Total
Drug use								
				Acculturation				
No	93.7	90.2	75.9	85.7	98.4	93.1	86.2	93.4
Yes	6.3	9.8	24.1	14.3	1.6	6.9	13.8	6.6

$N = 446, r = .21, p < .001$ $N = 638, r = .20, p < .001$

				Traditionalism A				
No	81.8	85.2	88.1	85.7	91.3	93.0	96.5	93.4
Yes	18.2	14.8	11.9	14.3	8.7	7.0	3.5	6.6

$N = 446, r = -.09, p < .05$ $N = 638, r = -.10, p < .05$

[a]Acculturation and traditionalism A grouped into discrete categories for the purpose of presentation. Correlations were obtained from unrecoded versions of the variables.
[b]Numbers are percents.

the prior 12 months (8.7% vs. 3.5%) while males with low traditionalism also were more likely to use drugs as those scoring high on traditionalism (18.2% vs. 11.9%) (see Table 6.6).

A SUMMARY OF ACCULTURATION AND TRADITIONALISM (A) CORRELATIONS WITH OUTCOMES

In sum, when we compare the correlations between acculturation and traditionalism and the outcomes (see Tables 6.1–6.6) we find that these impact men and women differently. Acculturation is significantly correlated with all of the outcome variables for males except for level of drinking, while for females a significant correlation was found in only two of the outcomes: alcohol use (abstainer vs. drinker) and drug use. Specifically, we find that:

1. As the level of acculturation increased, so did the likelihood of being a drinker and/or a drug user for both males and females.
2. As the level of acculturation increased, so did the extent of drinking in different places for males.
3. As the level of acculturation increased, the likelihood of drinking problems decreased for men but not for women (acculturation appears to increase the extent of drinking in different settings for men, while seemingly providing the conditions in which it is done more responsibly).

Traditionalism A was correlated as follows:
1. As traditionalism increased, the likelihood of being a drinker and the extent of drinking in different places decreased for women.
2. As traditionalism increased, so did the number of problems for men.
3. The higher the traditionalism, the less the likelihood of using drugs for both men and women.

The idea of traditionalism as a substance misuse and abuse prophylaxis is readily apparent for women. In addition to reducing the likelihood of drug use, it also appears to decrease the likelihood of problems due to drinking. With the exception of employment and antisocial behaviors (both nonsignificant), as the level of traditionalism increases among women the likelihood and extent of engaging in the different unwanted outcome behaviors decrease.

RELIGIOSITY AND FATALISM

Two other areas that often are assumed to be related to Puerto Rican traditionalism are the strong currents of religion and fatalism that run through the island culture and continue on the mainland. Both of these spiritually based value systems are strong in the Puerto Rican culture and often are cited among those important factors that physical and mental health providers should understand and perhaps utilize when providing services to Hispanics for a number of conditions (Castro & Gutierres, 1997; Congress, 1990; Cuadrado, 1998; Domino, Fragoso, & Moreno, 1991; Gloria & Peregoy, 1996; Montijo, 1975; Neff & Hoppe, 1993; Purdy, Simari, & Colon, 1983; Rosado, 1980; Ruef, Litz, & Schlenger, 2000; Sandoval & De la Roza, 1986; Singer, 1984; Suchman, 1967). As many of the researchers have indicated, the complex dynamics of the relationship of religion and fatalism to the Puerto Rican culture and the dynamics of this upon substance use outcomes needs to be considered and if possible incorporated as part of the treatment modalities offered to clients.

What effect do religiosity and a fatalistic outlook have on substance abuse outcomes? We found that as the respondents level of religiosity increased, their likelihood of being a drinker, extent of drinking, and their use of illicit drugs decreased regardless of gender. The strength of the curbing impact of religiosity for males and females was similar with the exception of extent of drinking where the correlation for females was almost twice as large as that for males and illicit drug use where the strength of the relationship was three times greater for males than females (see Table 6.7). Religiosity, though, was positively related to a greater number of problems in the health area among the males, but not so for the females. This is not to suggest that religion is the producer of these health problems but rather that one's health-related alcohol problems may move men more toward their own religion as a substitute for the spirituality of Alcoholics Anonymous. For many linguistic and other cultural reasons, Alcoholics Anonymous has not been very appealing to the Hispanic male and even less so for Hispanic females (Hoffman, 1994; Tonigan, Connors, & Miller, 1998).

The role of fatalism can be of great importance in studies of Hispanic populations. A fatalistic view of life has been found to increase the level of stress for Hispanics (Neff, 1993; Nespor, 1985; Ross, Mirowsky, & Cockerham, 1983; Wheaton, 1983) and alcohol has been found to be a buffer against this stress, particularly among males (Neff, 1993). Significant relationships between fatalism and outcome variables were only found for the males. As the level of fatalism increased, so did the number of alcohol problems as a whole, the number of loss of control and antisocial behavior problems, and the likelihood of using illegal drugs. This finding confirms those made by other researchers studying fatalism and substance use (Natera, Herrejon, & Casco, 1988; Neff, 1993; Olmstead, Guy, O'Mally, & Bentler, 1991). The gist of these arguments is that persons who feel that their control over their own lives is minimal may not view substance use as one of the main elements of their destructive behavior leading to problems—an overriding *que sera, sera* attitude. This may be reflected in the correlation between fatalism and number of drinking problems for men (.14, $p < .01$).

TABLE 6.7. Correlations between Outcomes, Degree of Religiosity, and
Fatalism for Males and Females

Outcomes	Religiosity		Fatalism	
	Male	Female	Male	Female
Drinkers (male = 432; female = 635)	-.15**	-.18***	-.03	-.02
Level of Drinking (male = 284; female = 290)	-.12*	-.20**	-.07	.06
Extent of Drinking in Different Settings (male = 263; female = 248)	-.11	-.01	-.01	-.07
No. of Drinking Problems (male = 339; female = 299)	.10	-.03	.14**	.05
Problem Areas (male = 339; female = 299)				
Family and social	.07	-.00	.09	.06
Employment	.05	-.10	.04	-.04
Health	.16**	.00	.10	.05
Loss of control	.10	-.03	.16**	.02
Anti-social behavior	.01	-.09	.13*	.08
Illicit Drug use last year (male = 446; female = 638)	-.24***	-.08*	.11*	.04

* $p < .05$;   ** $p < .01$;   *** $p < .001$.

Among the types of problems also related to higher levels of fatalism were antisocial behavior problems involving arguments and fights with others. Other researchers have shown that fatalism or high levels of external locus of control is related to similar aggressive behavior among adolescents (Dykeman, Daehlin, Doyle, Flamer, & Theodore, 1996) and married couples (Theodore, 1992).

COMPARISON OF TRADITIONALISM INDICES AMONG
MARRIED RESPONDENTS

As discussed in Chapter 3, the traditionalism indices of Behavior and
Decision Making cannot be combined with Traditionalism A (attitude)
for an even stronger and more representative Index of Traditionalism
due to their restriction to a subgroup of the sample: those living in a
couple relationship. For future research, it would be worthwhile to
include questions tapping these dimensions of traditional behavior and
decision making for all marital statuses in the general populations of the
various Hispanic groups instead of formulating them for use only with
couples.

Nevertheless, it is still possible to compare how the behavioral and
decision-making indices, as well as the attitudes index, fared on these
outcomes for those 408 respondents who are married or cohabiting. Are
the indices consistent or contradictory?

In Table 6.8 we find that there is little differentiating the impact of
the three traditionalism indices when we look at the outcome variables,
but there are a few exceptions. Earlier (see Table 6.3) we found that as
the level of traditionalism (A) increased among all male drinkers so did
the likelihood of having at least one problem with drinking ($r = .16$, $p <$
.01). We do not find this among the married male drinkers, perhaps
because the stereotypic bravado that is embedded in *machismo* and
attributed to the traditional Puerto Rican man is replaced with the lesser
known *macho* attributes of *el caballero*, the supportive gentleman who is a
family protector and a gentleman—a good family man. For many men,
the desire to drink "with the boys" now clashes with their commitments
to their family. Following a similar line of reasoning we find when
examining Traditionalism D (Decision Making) that married females as
well (who are in more traditional households) are less likely to have any
drinking problem ($r = -.29$, $p < .05$) than was true for all females in the

TABLE 6.8. Correlations between Outcomes, Traditionalism A (Attitudes), Traditionalism B (Behavior), and Traditionalism D (Decision Making) for Married or Cohabiting Males and Females

Outcomes	Traditionalism A		Traditionalism B		Traditionalism D	
	Male	Female	Male	Female	Male	Female
Drinkers	-.11	-.14	.04	-.14	-.11	-.10
Level of drinking	-.02	-.11	.04	.08	.01	.10
Extent of drinking in different Settings	-.17*	-.20	.05	.19	-.18*	-.18
Number of drinking problems	.08	-.13	-.03	.07	.03	-.29*
Problem Areas						
Family and social	.01	-.14	-.03	.09	-.00	-.23
Employment	.12	Insuff.	.01	Insuff.	.07	Insuff.
Health	.12	-.16	.00	.05	.07	-.20
Loss of control	.07	-.10	-.06	.08	.04	-.32**
Antisocial behavior	.05	-.12	-.03	.05	-.03	-.35**
Illicit drug use last year	-.13*	-.07	-.10	-.09	.05	-.08

$* p < .05;$ $** p < .01;$ $*** p < .001.$

sample ($r = -.06$, $p > .05$, see Table 6.3). In particular, for these married women, traditionalism, measured by male dominated decision making, provides the most protection from "loss of control" ($r = -.32$, $p < .01$) and "antisocial behaviors" ($r = -.35$, $p < .01$), both dangerous areas for the Puerto Rican woman who is looking after her family. Neither item was found to be significant for the female group as a whole in the sample (cf. Table 6.5).

With few exceptions, there is relative consistency among the three indices for the married and cohabiting group. We believe this reflects a higher level of abstraction, a more traditional outlook on life, a traditional *Weltanschauung,* which includes within it a set of cohesive traditional family values.

CHAPTER 7

A TYPOLOGY OF INTEGRATION

Puerto Ricans living on the mainland vary on the two dimensions of acculturation and traditionalism. These reflect different degrees of integration into mainstream (Anglo) culture. What can we learn from the construction of representative types based on different lifestyles of integration? What are the main demographic characteristics of those persons categorized into each of these types? How do these types relate to the substance misuse and abuse outcomes?

CREATING A TYPOLOGY OF INTEGRATION

We have examined and discussed the impacts that acculturation and traditionalism separately have on outcome situations. In actuality, different levels of acculturation and traditionalism are found simultaneously in each person. While it may be "common sense" to assume that those who are scored "high" on acculturation will likely be "low" on traditionalism, this may not necessarily be the case. As we have noted in Chapter 3, the correlation between the indices of acculturation and traditionalism A was relatively low ($r = -.29$, $p < .001$) given the common sense expectation that low traditionalism should be a function of high acculturation. This means that respondents may be found to be ranked "high" on both acculturation and traditionalism while others scored "low" on both indices. If we consider the several types that may emerge from combining both adaptations, we may construct four possible types by dividing each continuum at the median score (see Table 7.1) (for a discussion regarding types and uses of typologies, see Babbie, 1989; Barton, 1955; Rosenberg, 1968).

Type 1 represents a hypothetical construct of persons who are relatively highly acculturated and relatively lacking in manifesting the traditional ways of their culture of origin. In the minds of large numbers of Americans, this type represents the older pre-1950s notion of the successful immigrant—the product of the early 20th century concept of the "melting pot." The phrase was coined by Israel Zangwill, a Jew from England, who marveled at the tremendous influx of European immigrants to America at the beginning of the century. Zangwill's (1913) play *The Melting Pot* embodied a belief that all these newcomers would be transformed into new "Americans" and be undifferentiated from the older Americans with whom they would share the same language, values, and culture. This assimilation of the newcomers and their

TABLE 7.1. Model for Typology Construction: Acculturation by Traditionalism

	Acculturation	
	High	Low
Traditionalism		
Low	Type 1	Type 2
High	Type 3	Type 4

children, including those born in the United States was at times severely carried out using the instrumentality of the schools and government agencies. In the personal experience of one of the authors of this volume, children attending public schools in New York City in the late 1930s were made to feel ashamed if their parents had not yet learned English and were penalized for any expression of "old country" mannerisms and interests: European colloquialisms, musical tastes, food, accent, clothing, and so forth. In a sense, the ideal was to become fully acculturated and leave behind all traces of European traditions and superstitions; in other words, to become a "thoroughly modern American." It is this type of person who we believe is defined in cell 1 in Table 7.1, and we therefore label this type "The Moderns." Some of the aspirations of immigrants who wanted to quickly reach these goals and the often humorous consequences, especially on English language usage, was reflected in the classic *The Education of H*Y*M*A*N K*A*P*L*A*N*, originally published in 1937 (Rosten, 1965).

In the decades after World War II, with the rise of the civil rights movement and the numerous ethnic, gender, age, and other self-designated "power movements," American subgroups began to redefine themselves and their relationships to move more toward cultural pluralism not merely as a *de facto* recognition as pointed out by Glazer and Moynihan (1963) in *Beyond the Melting Pot*, but more importantly as having *de jure* standing with an emphasis on diversity being positive not only for the ethnic and other groups involved but for the nation as a whole. Although a full acceptance and understanding of the meaning and limits of cultural pluralism and diversity is still in the process of development, the public arena and discussion has been opened to the development and legitimacy of models other than that represented by "The Moderns."

Type 4 describes another extreme: those ethnic group members who resist integration and assimilation and adapt their lifestyle to minimally depart from their culture of origin. They do not learn the English language to any degree of fluency, restrict their social interactions to others of their own ethnicity, maintain food, music, and even medical care by limiting their choice of involvements as much as possible to only those in their ethnic group. They are usually found living in communities that are homogeneous and orient their personal goals to the communities from which they (or their parents) came. New values and change are often threatening and resisted, especially those affecting their children. Many believe that they will return to the places from which they came and their functioning here is to facilitate that return. This belief in their return is often the driving force behind the resistance to adapt through integration (Berry, 1980). These, in Cell 4, we have called "The Old-Worlders."

In characterizing the two remaining cells in this typology we find:

1. Type 2 persons who are not very acculturated to the "American way of life" and yet have abandoned or lost commitment to traditional cultural involvements and expressions.
2. Type 3, their opposite counterparts—persons who are very integrated into the American core culture and are also very much attached to their culture of origin.

Type 2 persons, who are ranked low on both acculturation and traditionalism, are the most difficult to conceptualize. To move away from one's culture and to abandon those values and role definitions learned since childhood is not likely to occur without a concomitant movement toward an alternative. It is during this transitory stage that the immigrant attempts to integrate into this new culture (which has not yet been sufficiently learned and internalized for adequate functioning), but may not have maintained a strong safety net of identity with the previous patterns of tradition. This may best be characterized by Schutz's (1944) concept of The Stranger, someone who has consciously abandoned his old identity and is attempting to fit into a new culture as a total lifestyle but who has not yet reached linguistic and social competence. In a sense, they have become the "Rootless."

Until recently, the goals of individuals coming to America was to become as Americanized as quickly as possible: someone who would be scored as "high" on acculturation and as "low" on traditionalism (i.e., adherence to the ways of the culture of origin) as possible. The ideal was to leave the old ways behind, but the person who was trapped somewhere in the middle of this transition was viewed as laden with internal strife and stress and as being *marginal* to the rest of the society. It is not surprising, therefore, that a large amount of the literature on the phenomenon of living in two cultures at the same time has focused on the negative consequences of this middle state (depression, anxiety, loneliness, etc.) (Arrowood, 1979; Cortes, Rogler, & Malgady, 1994; LaFromboise, Coleman, & Gerton, 1993; Ramirez & Hosch, 1991; Valdez, 2000). These persons also have been termed "low-level biculturals" (Felix-Ortiz, Newcomb, & Myers, 1994) or being in an "unsure stage" (Quiles, 1989) and are not the conceptual opposites of those in type 3 but may in fact be in transition to this adaptation.

If the "Moderns" represent an ethnic group goal that has lost its viability and appeal to more recent immigrant groups, the ethos implicit in type 3 may be the basis for the new ethnic identities. Persons who scored high on acculturation *and* high on traditionalism appear, on the surface to have the best chances for successful adaptation to the Anglo core culture without the sacrifices of loss of ethnic identity and pride. Indeed, recent research with Hispanics has found that the two-world behaviors and attitudes of these "Biculturals" provide a refuge for the stress of acculturation (Suarez, Fowers, Garwood, & Szapocznik, 1997). They defined biculturality as involving

> ...language and behavioral preferences, allowing the individual to feel comfortable in two diverse cultural environments. Biculturalism is seen as developing along two independent dimensions, one of which involves a linear process of accommodation to the host culture. The other dimension

involves a complex process by which an individual maintains some values
and attachments to the culture of origin and modifies others. (p. 491)

In Table 7.2, we present the distribution of types of integration
found in this sample. Table 7.2 does not purport to completely reflect the
distribution of types of integration within the mainland Puerto Rican
community, since the bifurcation process for reducing the scores of each
of the indices into approximately equal proportions does not represent
the only way of presenting and analyzing this data. For example, rather
than a dichotomy one might collapse the variables into a five-point scale
for each index. This would result in more stringently isolating the
extremes (the *most* highly acculturated and *least* traditional persons
found among The Moderns and the *least* acculturated and *most*
traditional among The Old-Worlders). These would theoretically
represent the expected placements if we assume that acculturation and
traditionalism should be inversely related. Weights could then be
assigned to each remaining "deviant case" cell, "...cases which do not
exhibit the behavior or the attitudes which we expected of them..."

TABLE 7.2. Types of Ethnic Group Adaptation

	Acculturation		
	High	Low	Total
Traditionalism			
	1. Moderns	2. Rootless	
Low	317	183	500
	(29.2%)	(16.9%)	
	3. Biculturals	4. Old-worlders	
High	236	348	584
	(21.8%)	(32.1%)	
Total	553	531	1084

$\chi^2(1, N = 1084) = 56.97, p < .001$.

(Kendall & Wolf, 1957, p. 167), in order to place them into one or another of the remaining two types. While perhaps more representative of the types at the extremes, this device would no more be representative of the community than the one we have chosen and would be less useful for statistical analyses and presentation of types. Suffice to say that any use of a typology is more for analytic than representative purposes.

BACKGROUND CHARACTERISTICS OF INTEGRATION TYPES

A major focus of analysis in drinking and substance use patterns maintained in this volume is that of the relationship of gender to other variables. In Table 7.3, we present the distribution of males and females for in each integration type.

Women were almost twice as likely to be Rootless as men (20.8% vs. 11.2%) and men were almost twice as likely as women to be Biculturals (29.8% vs. 16.1%). Both findings reflect the fact of a greater likelihood of males going out into the Anglo community for work and other business

TABLE 7.3. Distribution of Respondents in Typology of Integration

Typology classification	Male		Female	
	N	%	N	%
Moderns (high acculturation /low traditionalism)	121	27.1	196	30.7
Rootless (low acculturation /low traditionalism)	50	11.2	133	20.8
Biculturals (high acculturation /high traditionalism)	133	29.8	103	16.1
Old-worlders (low acculturation/high traditionalism)	142	31.8	206	32.3
Total	446	100.0	638	100.0

$\chi^2(3, N = 1084) = 38.16, p < .001.$

than women are. In Table 7.4, we present the correlations between the demographic variables and the typology separately for males and females.

In brief, what are the modal characteristics of each type?

1. The Moderns are more likely to be female, persons born in mainland United States or who came to the United States at a mean age of 11, high school graduates or beyond, employed, with a reported income mostly above $15,000, and a mean age of 33.

2. The Rootless are more likely to be female, persons born in Puerto Rico or who came to the United States at a mean age of 23, did not go to high school, more homemakers than employed, a reported income mostly below $8,000, and a mean age of 48.

3. The Biculturals are more likely to be male, persons born in Puerto Rico or who came to the United States at a mean age of 12, some high school education, mostly employed, a reported income above $10,000, and a mean age of 36.

4. The Old-Worlders are more likely to be female, born in Puerto Rico and came to the United States at a mean age of 25, did not go to high school, equally employed or homemakers, a reported income mostly less than $6,000, and a mean age of 51.

As shown in Table 7.4, there are striking similarities for the modal categories between males and females found in all of the types with the exception of marital status and employment. Married males are more likely to be "Old-Worlders" and married females mostly found among the "Moderns." Employed males were more likely to be found among the "Biculturals" and employed women among the "Moderns."

Table 7.4. Demographic Characteristics of Respondents in Typology of Integration by Gender[a]

	Male				Female			
	Rootless (N=50)	Old-worlders (N=142)	Moderns (N=121)	Biculturals (N=133)	Rootless (N=133)	Old-worlders (N=206)	Moderns (N=196)	Biculturals (N=103)
Born in Puerto Rico	15.8	43.0	16.1	25.1	26.3	42.7	19.3	11.7
Married	11.0	35.2	26.1	27.7	22.6	24.0	36.3	17.1
Completed high school or more	5.5	12.6	44.5	37.4	15.2	14.8	53.0	17.0
Employed	10.6	28.4	29.4	31.6	15.2	21.7	46.3	16.8
Income ($6000 or less)	8.0	48.0	18.0	26.0	21.2	42.0	21.8	15.0
Mean age at interview	50.7	52.2	33.0	36.9	47.2	50.8	33.5	35.8
Mean age to United States (for those born in Puerto Rico)	24.2	25.8	13.6	12.0	23.1	24.3	9.7	12.1

[a]Percentaged on demographics.

THE SIMULTANEOUS EFFECTS OF ACCULTURATION AND TRADITIONALISM ON OUTCOME VARIABLES

Among the goals of this study is to examine the influence that the addition of a high level of traditionalism will have on the negative effects of acculturation on drinking and drug use outcomes. We believe that the findings may be useful for development or enhancement of social action programs in these areas for Puerto Ricans. Consideration of the suitability for intervention with either the acculturation process or traditionalism attitudes suggests that the variable that most likely can be influenced to prevent or mitigate the likelihood of occurrence of outcomes is traditionalism. Acculturation could only be realistically influenced by accelerating the process but, it has been found by others and confirmed by this study that greater acculturation is linked to greater harmful involvement in many of the outcome activities (alcohol use, alcohol problems, and drug use). It is our contention, supported by the data in this study, that an "increase in traditionalism" may mitigate many of the negative effects of becoming highly acculturated. Traditionalism may be safely manipulated, since it can involve a sense of pride for the Puerto Rican culture, attachment to values that make the family important, and curtail culturally inappropriate behavior among other dimensions by drawing on and emphasizing not the limiting and sometimes destructive elements of *marianismo* and *machismo* but the positive aspects of *hembrismo* (a concept exalting the strength and survival abilities of indigenous Puerto Rican women) and the *caballero* (the supportive husband, family man, and gentleman).

In order to examine the impact of traditionalism on the outcome variables for the more highly acculturated Puerto Rican, four dichotomous dummy variables consisting of each of the types (yes/no) were created. Table 7.5 presents Pearson correlations for each type and the outcome variables:

TABLE 7.5. Correlations between Outcomes and Typology of Integration by Gender

	Males				Females			
	Rootless (LT/LA)[a]	Old-worlders (HT/LA)	Moderns (LT/HA)	Biculturals (HT/HA)	Rootless (LT/LA)	Old-worlders (HT/LA)	Moderns (LT/HA)	Biculturals (HT/HA)
Drinkers	-.10*	-.08	.13**	.02	-.12**	-.17***	.16***	.14***
Level of drinking	.06	.01	.04	-.08	.07	-.15*	.07	.01
Extent (different places)	-.01	-.15*	.15*	-.01	.01	-.13*	.16*	-.07
Number of alcohol problems	.05	.21***	-.14**	-.10	.02	-.03	.03	-.02
Family	.07	.14*	-.13*	-.06	-.02	-.04	.01	.04
Employment	.03	.12*	.08	-.07	.05	-.06	-.08	.11
Health	.07	.16**	-.13*	-.08	.01	-.04	.08	-.05
Loss of control	.11*	.14**	-.17**	-.05	-.07	.03	.04	-.02
Antisocial behavior	.02	.11*	-.06	-.07	.02	-.07	.01	.04
Drug use	-.06	-.14**	.10*	.10*	-.09*	-.12**	.17***	.04

$*$ $p < .05$; $**$ $p < .01$; $***$ $p < .001$.

[a] LT, low traditionalism; HT, high traditionalism; LA, low acculturation; HA, high acculturation.

1. Drinkers: In mainland United States, high acculturation seems to overpower any effects that high traditionalism might have in inhibiting the choice of drinking or not, especially for women. For women, both high acculturation types (Moderns and Biculturals) were more likely to contain drinkers than the low acculturation types (Rootless and Old-Worlders), irrespective of the presence of high traditionalism. Within the two high acculturation types, the presence of high traditionalism only negligibly decreases the likelihood of female abstinence, but it does appear to nullify the impact of high acculturation for men.

2. Level of drinking: For men, as we found earlier in Table 6.2, neither acculturation nor traditionalism affects level of drinking. In Table 7.5, we find that combining high traditionalism with acculturation still does not produce a significant effect. For women, the only significant outcome reflects the stereotype of the traditional Puerto Rican woman: one who is high on tradition and low on acculturation (Old-Worlders). There was no effect of traditionalism on the high acculturation types (Moderns and Biculturals).

3. Extent of drinking in different places: Traditionalism has an important role to play for both men and women in reducing the extent of drinking in different places. When traditionalism is high and acculturation is Low (Old-Worlders), there is a decrease in extent of drinking and vice versa (Moderns).

4. Number of alcohol problems and problem types: There were no significant correlations between total number of alcohol problems (or problem types) and the typology for females. We have seen, however, that acculturation appears to be beneficial to males regarding problem drinking (see Table 6.5), that is, high acculturation reduces the likelihood of problems. In Table 7.5, we find that traditionalism when combined with acculturation provides interesting aspects of the meaning of traditionalism for men. For the three alcohol-related problem areas of family, health and loss of control, males in the two high acculturation

groups (Moderns and Biculturals) exhibited less of a tendency to manifest problems in these areas than those in the low acculturation groups. It appears also that increased tradition does little or may even have a deleterious effect on men who scored higher on acculturation (Biculturals compared to Moderns) in these three problem areas. This is reinforced by comparing the Rootless and the Old-Worlders where we find that the presence of high traditionalism (Old-Worlders) increases the likelihood of having problems in all the areas. Why should this be so? As we have pointed out in several places in this volume, for many Hispanic males a highly traditional outlook may mean for them to have license to engage in alcohol excesses. While high traditionalism may affect external patterns of drinking with respect to abstinence, level of drinking, and extent in different settings, the Puerto Rican males seem to have difficulty controlling the *consequences* of drinking in a society that is less tolerant of drunkenness among males. If traditionalism is a positive force to be increased in prevention and treatment programs, emphasis on the negative consequences of drinking seems much more important for the males than for the females even for the highly acculturated males.

5. Drug use: For both men and women, those in high acculturation groups (Moderns and Biculturals) were more likely to use drugs than those in low acculturation groups. For women, however, the presence of high traditionalism among the Biculturals nullifies the likelihood of using drugs. This is not true for the men. When we compare males who are Moderns and Biculturals (high acculturation types) versus the Rootless and Old-Worlders (low acculturation types) we find no benefits of a higher traditionalism for the Biculturals over the Moderns but a significant decrease for the Old-Worlders over the Rootless.

CHAPTER 8

ETHNOTHERAPY IMPLICATIONS
AND CONCLUSIONS

In this volume we have analyzed a sample of the mainland Puerto Rican population to examine and test the proposition that a general loss of traditional family values—measured by gender-related values of the roles and behavior of family members—may contribute to the specific albeit unrelated deviant outcomes of alcohol and drug use. More specifically, we have contended that it is not necessarily the adherence to or lack of *specific* regulatory norms that may affect drug and alcohol use behaviors of Puerto Ricans in mainland United States, but rather adherence to or rejection of a general commitment to Hispanic values. This we have called "traditionalism," particularly as it relates to the definitions of gender role behavior of Puerto Rican men and women. These values had once served, for women, as a brake or control mechanism on substance misuse. While many researchers, who have studied drug and alcohol abuse among Hispanics, including Puerto Ricans, have suggested acculturation alone as the explanation for changing substance use patterns of these Hispanics in the United States, we have attempted to demonstrate that rather, it is the movement away

181

from "traditionalism" itself that effects an increase in substance misuse and abuse.

The conclusions reached in this volume reflect the view that despite the social rhetoric of the past decade, it is not the absence of specific proscriptive values alone that must be rectified to prevent certain individual and social ills but rather it is the promotion of a "sense of tradition" itself that is needed. This sense of tradition can best be derived from the pride and knowledge about one's ethnic group, for it is *ethnic pride and identification* that may provide, to paraphrase the psychologist Kurt Lewin (1948), "a firm ground on which to stand," i.e., a strong bond linking one's self through the family to a larger community. Individual and interpersonal choices, often emotionally compelling, may then be made with respect to one's ethnic community reference group. It is the strength of the ties to the culture of origin and its traditions that allows the immigrant to resist the stresses of acculturation that might otherwise result in their being vulnerable to substance use as a means of coping.

In our separate analyses of the impact that acculturation and traditionalism have on the use of alcohol and drugs among Puerto Ricans, as well as when the simultaneous effects of these factor were examined, we found that acculturation and traditionalism do not affect men and women in the same way. For males we found that as the level of acculturation increased so did the likelihood of: (1) being a drinker (regardless of the level of traditionalism), (2) the extent of drinking in different places (with higher traditionalism tempering this effect), and (3) being a drug user (with traditionalism not affecting the impact of acculturation). The level of drinking among men was not affected by either acculturation or traditionalism, even when these factors were combined.

Acculturation was found to have a preventive role to play in inhibiting the development of male alcohol problems but the opposite effect is true for traditionalism where we found that the greater the traditionalism, the greater the likelihood of problems (which we attribute to greater community and peer group tolerance of problems among more traditional men). The problematic drinking areas for men with low acculturation and high traditionalism were family, health, and loss of control. However, we found that traditionalism did not increase the likelihood of drinking problems among those with more responsibilities, namely, the married male drinkers. This may be due to the cultural fact that when a man marries and has children other elements of the male role surface and take precedence over the carefree single male behavior. These elements are those of *el caballero*, the family provider and protector. An increase in these elements of traditionalism for men would appear to be warranted.

Among the women, the higher the level of acculturation the likelier they were: (1) to be drinkers (regardless of the level of traditionalism), (2) to drink at a higher extent in a number of different settings (although this effect of acculturation was reduced by higher levels of traditionalism, and (3) to have used drugs (however, the presence of high traditionalism was found to nullify the likelihood of using drugs among highly acculturated women). For female drinkers, neither acculturation nor traditionalism was correlated with problem drinking in any of the areas examined. In brief, *a more traditional outlook appears to have clear and positive benefits for women by decreasing the likelihood of problematic alcohol and drug use and misuse irrespective of level of acculturation.*

An inference that one might draw from the findings in this study is that the traditional *marianismo* passive–submissive role has desirable qualities for women and should be enhanced, while the *macho* dominant role is not and should not be strengthened. We believe that both inferences would be incorrect and unwise. Our reasoning for this is simple. Both roles contain many more elements that frequently are unrecognized and lie dormant. These elements also are part of Hispanic "tradition" and may be emphasized to achieve the positive benefits of traditionalism for both men and women. We refer to the elements within *hembrismo* for women and *el caballero* for men.

The mechanism that we suggest for positive change in these gender roles is "ethnotherapy." The term, "ethnotherapy," is usually attributed to a psychiatrist Price Cobbs who first applied it to problems of black identity and their role in racial confrontation. Essentially, it was a clinical model to alter negative attitudes about one's own ethnic group and others as well, by exploring one's own feelings in this area. His therapy groups of blacks and whites sought to deepen the understanding that each had of the other. He believed that building a stronger and healthier ethnic self-identity would lessen the anger and hostility one had toward one's own ethnic group and toward others. Cobbs' (1972) work was expanded by a participant in one of his groups, Judith Weinstein Klein, who concentrated on the self-identity dimension and the problems related to poor and confused ethnic self-identity in one's relationship with one's own ethnic group. Klein focused on a Jewish population and the efficacy of a clinical group therapy in which feelings, attitudes, and behaviors concerning one's ethnic identity was the main subject of discussion and analyses (Klein, 1976, 1980). Other researchers and therapists also have examined the usefulness of ethnotherapy as an adjunct modality (Comas-Diaz & Jacobsen, 1987; Mann, 1987; Mirage, 1987; Ruiz, 1984; Terrell, 1993).

The findings presented in this volume are consistent with the suggestion that ethnotherapy may be used as an ancillary treatment modality for substance abuse as well as a prevention mechanism in this area for Puerto Rican and other ethnic groups. This emphasis on a return to tradition and traditional values does not place emphasis on the nonfunctional and discarded elements of any particular tradition but rather draws from the ego-enhancing elements already existing in that culture. For example, among Puerto Rican males, the emphasis would be away from the destructive aspects of *machismo* and toward the positive images of the traditional *caballero*, the supportive gentleman. Similarly, for women, the outmoded (and for some, destructive) syndrome of *marianismo* (submissiveness toward males and passive acceptance of destiny) may be replaced by *la nueva marianista*, the assertive and independent woman. This is a role proposed by Gil and Vazquez (1996) based on the constructive and supportive elements of the Hispanic wife and mother that draws on the traditional concept of *hembrismo* to be the basis of a different set of traditional family values that may be positive and productive even for the acculturated woman. *Hembrismo* has been described by Comas-Diaz (1987) in the following manner:

> Contemporary Puerto Rican women have begun to explore alternative roles. *Hembrismo*, which literally means femaleness, is one such attempt. The concept of *hembrismo* has historical roots, in that the Taino Indians, the indigenous Puerto Ricans, were a matriarchal society. Borinquén (Puerto Rico's Indian name) was ruled by the "earth mother," imbuing the female political influence with spiritual power....In addition, the advent of Black slavery on the island contributed to a basis for *hembrismo* in that the Black women, doubly oppressed by gender and race, needed to develop strength for survival and flexibility for adaptation. Thus, *hembrismo* connotes strength, perseverance, flexibility, and an ability for survival. Mainland Puerto Rican women may adhere to the *hembrista* norm as a means of preserving their identity and cultural beliefs while simultaneously creating a more flexible role for themselves in American society. (p. 464).

Similarly, the role of *el macho* is not only defined by the hard-drinking womanizer, but also the responsible protector of home and family, the gentleman, *el caballero*. This concept, related to traditional views of *machismo*, belies the notion that a man must necessarily be "hard-drinking" in order to be respected by other men because it also contains the notion of *indecente*, the type of drinking behavior resulting in drunkenness that thus would be termed "undignified" (Johnson & Matre, 1978).

In order to accomplish these alterations in the mind-set of Puerto Rican women and men as part of the process of treatment or prevention of alcohol and other substance abuse, some elaboration of the issues involved in ethnotherapy with this population is necessary. We are not suggesting that ethnotherapy is to be considered as a treatment modality in itself, but rather as an ancillary treatment tool to help in a resocialization process geared to alter perception and acceptance of gender role definitions and behaviors in the direction of a more positive traditionalism perspective. We believe that using an ethnotherapeutic approach can be useful with therapeutic communities, group therapies, individual patient–therapist relationships, peer group sessions, religious settings, 12-step programs such as Alcoholics Anonymous, or whatever combinations are available. Our expectation is that ethnotherapy as described here will benefit clients and patients in all settings to be better able to handle the stresses of acculturation and maladaptation.

GOALS OF ETHNOTHERAPY WITH HISPANICS

The goals for patients and clients in different ethnic groups, of necessity, will be different and need to be clarified and understood by staff and clients so that methods and concepts used will constitute a cohesive whole. The first goal to be achieved is the ethnocultural identification between the client and the therapist. It is the *sine qua non* of all other goals and methods. Comas-Diaz and Jacobsen (1987) have emphasized the use of ethnocultural identification in psychotherapy:

> Ethnocultural identification is a therapeutic process that fosters an identification in which the therapist reflects pieces of the patient's ethnocultural self. It supports patients' identification with the therapist and thereby helps to create a foundation for beginning the work of reconstructing a fragmented identity. (p. 236)

A difficulty with the implementation of this goal that staff need to be aware of is the reality of the cultural differences not only in settings composed of persons from different Hispanic groups but also differences in acculturation and traditionalism levels, especially groups mixed with Old-Worlders and Moderns. Other goals should also include:

1. Creating an accepting rather than confrontational environment.
2. Heightening ethnic pride and identity (vital for Hispanic group members that still face discrimination and stereotyped responses by the Anglo communities).
3. Reduce acculturation stress.
4. Alter role self definitions based more on *hembrismo* and *el caballero*.

TECHNIQUES OF ETHNOTHERAPY

The methods of ethnotherapy with Hispanic groups need not be complicated and can be adapted for use in the context of a variety of treatment modalities. They are of necessity specific to the particular Hispanic group considered. The following are some of the techniques used by therapists:

1. "Ethnicize" the physical and institutional space as well as the activities within the space, for example, motifs, pictures, music, celebration of holidays, dances, and food (Santiago-Irizarry, 1996).
2. During ethnotherapy sessions, focus on the ethnic issues in common among group members rather than on personal idiosyncratic nonethnic issues.
3. Use of language switching to allow clients to switch back and forth between Spanish and English, whichever is most comfortable for expression at the time (Altarriba & Santiago-Rivera, 1994; Delgado, 1998a; Santiago-Rivera, 1995).
4. Use of *dichos* (proverbs and folk sayings) as the focus of discussions. *Dichos* "describe attitudes, behaviors, and moral values" (Altarriba & Santiago-Rivera, 1994, p. 392): "A dicho is a popular saying expressing truth or folk wisdom and is generally symbolic...such as *Dime con quien andas y te dire quien eres* (Tell me

who your friends are and I can tell you who you are), and *A quien madruga, Dios lo ayuda* (God helps early risers), which often provide some comforting advice" (Santiago-Rivera, 1995, p. 14).

5. Enlisting the aid of Hispanic natural support systems such as the extended family members, neighbors, friends, healers, local self-help groups, community and religious leaders, as well as commercial establishments, *bodegas*, clothing stores, food establishments, and *botanicas* (herbal shops). All of these may serve to help in different personal and institutional ways, distribute information, and provide services (Delgado, 1998b).

6. Use of *espiritistas* (spiritualists) where appropriate, since Puerto Ricans as well as many other Hispanics see them as legitimate and trustworthy healers (Comas-Diaz, 1986, 1988; Delgado, 1977; Gloria & Peregoy, 1996; Singer, 1984).

CONTEXTUAL CONCEPTS

In the context of working with Hispanic clients and using an ethnotherapeutic orientation, certain concepts of importance to all Hispanic ethnic groups must be taken into consideration. These can help break down barriers between patient and therapist and provide psychological supports and insights to the healers and service providers as well as those we are attempting to help change. These are concepts that may have important ramifications whether raised during sessions as issues or not.

1. *Familismo*. While most Americans understand the importance of family, for Hispanics it takes on much stronger and emotional connotations. *Familismo* represents the strong bonds of loyalty, identity, and responsibility given to and expected from each member of a Hispanic family. It is the main source of identity as well as support. These strong bonds can exist even when members are not in contact with

each other and often survive the highest levels of acculturation. Members of a family are often measured by the pride (*respeto* and *dignidad*) or shame (*verguenza*) that he or she brings to the family (Canino & Canino, 1982; Comas-Diaz, 1993; Gloria & Peregoy, 1996; Rodriquez-Andrew, 1998; Sandoval & De la Roza, 1986; Vazquez-Nuttall et al., 1984).

2. *Personalismo*. Personalism is a Hispanic notion of close, friendly, familiar relationships between individuals. This is often a difficult gap to bridge for therapists who are trained to maintain role relationships with clients based on regulated expectations of the client and therapist roles. Movement outside the role confines to a personal relationship between counselor and patient is usually frowned on and sometimes considered unethical. *Personalismo* does not mean that the personal relationship exists outside of the therapy situation but that the Hispanic client is most comfortable and trusting when the therapist is also to be treated as a whole person and not merely as a role, just as the client expects himself or herself to be treated (Gloria & Peregoy, 1996; Sandoval & De la Roza, 1986).

3. *Fatalismo*. Fatalism has been defined as "the perception that there is no protection against adversity and that anything that happens to anybody can happen to me" (Sandoval & De la Roza, 1986, p. 174). Many Hispanics firmly believe that they are powerless to control their own future and that problems are to be accepted because they are God's will or "destiny" (Congress, 1990; Sandoval & De la Roza, 1986; Vazquez-Nuttall et al., 1984). Resistances to therapy by Hispanics due to their unconscious belief in *fatalismo* can be readily examined and dealt with in the context of ethnotherapy sessions.

4. *Respeto y verguenza*. The two notions of respect and shame are very strongly entwined in the Hispanic psyche. People are intrinsically owed respect and if someone behaves disrespectfully toward the family or others, he or she is acting in a shameful manner. To act in a shameful manner by drinking improperly or doing drugs is to bring shame not

only to one's self but, through this lack of respect shown for the family, to bring shame to the family. This notion of not showing respect to and for the family and bringing shame to them can be a powerful ally to help Hispanics change behavior. In one sense, it represents the positive use of guilt in a therapeutic setting. Counselors or psychotherapists who use ethnotherapy also should be aware that *verguenza* may be the basis for resistances to treatment. In order to avoid shame, families of substance abusers may isolate themselves. Through isolation, they will not have to reveal their problems to a stranger (service provider) and risk community awareness that they had reached outside of the family for help (Gloria & Peregoy, 1996).

This brief outline of ethnotherapy with Hispanics is merely a suggestion for creating a therapeutic and accepting environment in which Hispanic substance abusers can raise their levels of traditionalism and ethnic identity as a foundation for dealing with their substance abuse. It obviously is not meant to replace other more conventional medical and psychological modalities but to place them in a more meaningful context for Puerto Rican and other Hispanic clients. As the Hispanic population in the United States increases, especially at the rate of the last few years, we are likely to see more Hispanics in need of substance abuse treatment. We have found that an emphasis on a more traditional outlook for Puerto Ricans would be helpful in this problem area and a plausible antidote to some of the impacts of an inevitable acculturation process.

The value of tradition and the subjective meaning of the various components of tradition rather than adherence to specific traditional cultural norms are the key elements in our approach to ethnicity-based programs. It is the pride and commitment to one's tradition and family and not bringing shame to either that itself can be considered an ancillary treatment modality. This approach may be seen as a model to be built on in the various secular and Anglo communities of the wider populations for treatment of a variety of socially undesirable behaviors. They are an affirmation of the principle that conventional and conformist behaviors are more a product of internal mechanisms and conscience than external social controls.

REFERENCES

Aguirre-Molina, M. (1991). Issues for Latinas: Puerto Rican women. In P. Roth (Ed.), *Alcohol and drugs are women's issues: Review of issues* (pp. 93–100). Metuchen, NJ: Scarecrow Press.

Alcocer, A. (1977). *Final report of a study of drinking practices and alcohol-related problems of Spanish-speaking persons in three California locales.* Alhambra, CA: Technical Services Institute.

Alcocer, A. (1982). Alcohol use and abuse among the Hispanic American population. *In Special Populations Issue: Alcohol and Health* (pp. 367–382). Washington, DC: National Institute of Alcohol Abuse and Alcoholism.

Aleichem, S. (1956). *Selected stories of Sholom Aleichem.* New York: Modern Library.

Altarriba, J., & Santiago-Rivera, A. (1994). Current perspectives on using linguistic and cultural factors in counseling the Hispanic client. *Professional Psychology: Research & Practice, 25*(4), 388–397.

Amaro, H., Coffman, G., & Herren, T. (1990). Acculturation and marijuana and cocaine use findings from HHANES 1982–84. *American Journal of Public Health, 80,* 54–60.

Arredondo, R., Weddige, R. L., Justice, C. L., & Fitz, J. (1987). Alcoholism in Mexican–Americans: Intervention and treatment. *Hospital & Community Psychiatry, 38*(2), 180–183.

Arrowood, N. R. F. (1979). Problem: The use/abuse of drugs as an indicator of the bilingual/bicultural assimilation difficulties encountered by Mexican-

Americans coping with the Anglo-American mainstream--A literature review. ERIC Microfiche Number: ED186184.

Austin, G. A., & Gilbert, J. M. (1989). Substance abuse among Latino youth. *Prevention Research Update, 3*, 1–25.

Babbie, E. (1989). *The practice of social research* (5th ed.). Belmont, CA: Wadsworth.

Barton, A. H. (1955). The concept of property–space in social research. In P. F. Lazarsfeld & M. Rosenberg (Eds.), *The language of social research* (pp. 40–53). Glencoe, IL: Free Press.

Benson, H. (1975). *The relaxation response.* New York: Avon Books.

Berry, J. W. (1980). Acculturation as varieties of adaptation. In A. M. Padilla (Ed.), *Acculturation: Theory, models, and some new findings* (pp. 9–25). Boulder, CO: Westview Press for the Advancement of Science.

Black, S. A., & Markides, K. S. (1993). Acculturation and alcohol consumption in Puerto Rican, Cuban-American, and Mexican-American women in the United States. *American Journal of Public Health, 83*(6), 890–893.

Booth, M. W., Castro, F. G., & Anglin, M. D. (1990). What do we know about Hispanic substance abuse? A review of the literature. In R. Glick & J. Moore (Eds.), *Drugs in Hispanic communities* (pp. 21–43). New Brunswick, NJ: Rutgers University Press.

Byrd, T., Cohn, L. D., Gonzalez, E., Parada, M., & Cortes, M. (1999). Seatbelt use and belief in destiny among Hispanic and non-Hispanic drivers. *Accident Analysis & Prevention, 31*(1–2), 63–65.

Caetano, R. (1984a). Ethnicity and drinking in northern California: A comparison among whites, blacks, and Hispanics. *Alcohol & Alcoholism, 19*(1), 31–44.

Caetano, R. (1984b). Hispanic drinking practices in northern California. *Hispanic Journal of Behavioral Sciences, 6*(4), 345–364.

Caetano, R. (1985). Drinking patterns and alcohol problems in a national sample of US Hispanics, *In Alcohol use among US ethnic minorities: Proceedings of a conference on the epidemiology of alcohol use and abuse among ethnic minority groups. Research Monograph No. 18* (pp. 147–162.). Washington, DC: US Department of Health and Human Services.

Caetano, R. (1986). Alternative definitions of Hispanics: Consequences in an alcohol survey. *Hispanic Journal of Behavioral Sciences, 8*(4), 331–344.

Caetano, R. (1987a). Acculturation and drinking patterns among US Hispanics. *British Journal of Addiction, 82*(7), 789–799.

Caetano, R. (1987b). Acculturation, drinking and social settings among US Hispanics. *Drug and Alcohol Dependence, 19*(3), 215–226.

Caetano, R. (1988). Alcohol uses among Hispanic groups in the United States. *American Journal of Drug and Alcohol Abuse, 14*(3), 293-308.

Caetano, R., Clark, C., & Tam, T. (1998). Alcohol consumption among racial/ethnic minorities: Theory and research. *Alcohol Health and Research World, 22*(4), 233-241.

Caetano, R., & Medina Mora, M. E. (1988). Acculturation and drinking among people of Mexican descent in Mexico and the United States. *Journal of Studies on Alcohol, 49*(5), 462–471.

Cahalan, D., Cisin, Ira H., & Crossley, Helen M. (1969). *American Drinking Practices* (Vol. Monograph No. 6). New Brunswick, NJ: Rutgers Center of Alcohol Studies.

Campbell, P. R. (1996). *Population projections for states by age, sex, race, and Hispanic origin: 1995–2025*. Washington, DC: US Census Bureau, Population Projection Branch.

Canino, G. (1994). Alcohol use and misuse among Hispanic women: Selected factors, processes, and studies. Special issue: Substance use patterns of Latinas. *International Journal of the Addictions, 29*(9), 1083–1100.

Canino, G., Anthony, J. C., Freeman, D. H., Shrout, P., & Rubio-Stipec, M. (1993). Drug abuse and illicit drug use in Puerto Rico. *American Journal of Public Health, 83*(2), 194–200.

Canino, G., & Canino, I. A. (1982). Culturally syntonic family therapy for migrant Puerto Ricans. *Hospital and Community Psychiatry, 33*(4), 299-303.

Canino, G. J., Burnam, A., & Caetano, R. (1992). The prevalence of alcohol abuse and/or dependence in two Hispanic communities. In J. E. Helzer (Ed.), *Alcoholism in North America, Europe, and Asia* (pp. 131–155). New York: Oxford University Press.

Castro, F. G., & Gutierres, S. (1997). Drug and alcohol use among rural Mexican-Americans. In E. B. Robertson, Z. Sloboda, G. M. Boyd, L. Beatty, & N. J. Kozel (Eds.), *Rural substance abuse: State of knowledge and issues* (Vol. NIDA Research Monograph 168, pp. 498–530). Washington, DC: U.S. Department of Health and Human Services, National Institutes of Health.

Cervantes, R. C., Gilbert, J. M., Snyder, N. S., & Padilla, A. M. (1990–1991). Psychosocial and cognitive correlates of alcohol use in younger adult immigrants and US born Hispanics. *International Journal of the Addictions, 25,* 687–708.

Chafetz, M. E., & Demone, H. W. (1962). *Alcoholism and society.* New York: Oxford University Press.

Christensen, E. W. (1979). The Puerto Rican woman: A profile. In E. B. Acosta (Ed.), *The Puerto Rican woman* (pp. 51–63). New York: Praeger.

Cobbs, P. (1972). Ethnotherapy in groups. In L. Solomon & B. Berzon (Eds.), *New perspectives on encounter groups* (pp. 383-403). San Francisco: Jossey-Bass.

Comas-Diaz, L. (1986). Puerto Rican alcoholic women: Treatment considerations. *Alcoholism Treatment Quarterly, 3*(1), 47–57.

Comas-Diaz, L. (1987). Feminist therapy with mainland Puerto Rican women. *Psychology of Women Quarterly, 11,* 461–474.

Comas-Diaz, L. (1988). Mainland Puerto Rican women: A sociocultural approach. *Journal of Community Psychology, 16*(1), 21–31.

Comas-Diaz, L. (1989). Puerto Rican women's cross-cultural transitions: Developmental and clinical implications. In C. T. Garcia Cole & M. L. Mattei (Eds.), *The psychosocial development of Puerto Rican women* (pp. 166–199). New York: Praeger.

Comas-Diaz, L. (1993). Hispanic Latino communities: Psychological implications. In D. Atkinson, G. Morten, & D. W. Su (Eds.), *Counseling American minorities: A Cross-cultural perspective* (4th ed., pp. 245–263). Madison, WI: Brown & Benchmark.

Comas-Diaz, L., & Jacobsen, F. M. (1987). Ethnocultural identification in psychotherapy. *Psychiatry, 50*(August), 232–241.

Congress, E. P. (1990). Crisis intervention with Hispanic clients in an urban mental health clinic. In A. R. Roberts (Ed.), *Crisis intervention handbook: Assessment, treatment, and research* (pp. 221–236). Belmont, CA: Wadsworth Publishing Co.

Cortes, D. E., Rogler, L. H., & Malgady, R. G. (1994). Biculturality among Puerto Rican adults in the United States. *American Journal of Community Psychology, 22*(5), 707–721.

Cuadrado, M. (1997). *Social inhibitors of illicit drug use and problem drinking among Puerto Rican women.* Unpublished doctoral dissertation, City University of New York, New York.

Cuadrado, M. (1998). *Spiritualism and gambling*. Paper presented at the Florida Council on Compulsive Gambling Annual Conference, Orlando, Florida.

Cuadrado, M. (1999). Comparison of Hispanic and Anglo calls to a gambling help hotline. *Journal of Gambling Studies, 15*(1), 71–83.

Cuadrado, M., & Lieberman, L. (1998). Traditionalism in the prevention of substance misuse among Puerto Ricans. *Substance Use & Misuse, 33*(14), 2737–2755.

de Ortiz, S. A. (1981). *Alcoholism: Puerto Rican male and female social context of drinking patterns and their familistic ambiance*. Unpublished doctoral dissertation, Ohio State University, Columbus, OH.

Delgado, M. (1977). Puerto Rican spiritualism and the social work profession. *Social Casework, 58*(8), 451–458.

Delgado, M. (1998a). *Alcohol use/abuse among Latinos: Issues and examples of culturally competent services*. New York: Haworth Press.

Delgado, M. (1998b). *Social services in Latino communities: Research and strategies*. New York: Haworth Press.

Diaz, J. O. P., & Draguns, J. G. (1990). Mental health of two-way migrants: From Puerto Rico to the United States and return. *Migration World, XVIII* (3/4), 34–37.

Domino, G., Fragoso, A., & Moreno, H. (1991). Cross-cultural investigations of the imagery of cancer in Mexican nationals. *Hispanic Journal of Behavioral Sciences, 13*(4), 422–435.

Durkheim, E. (1951). *Suicide: A study in sociology* (J. A. Spaulding & G. Simpson, Trans.). Glencoe, IL: Free Press.

Durkheim, E. (1984). *The division of labor in society* (W. D. Halls, Trans.). New York: Free Press.

Dykeman, C., Daehlin, W., Doyle, S., Flamer, H. S., & Theodore, R. M. (1996). Psychological predictors of school-based violence: Implications for school counselors. *School Counselor, 44*(1), 35–47.

Estrada, A. (1982). Alcohol use among Hispanic adolescents: A preliminary report. *Hispanic Journal of Behavioral Sciences, 4*(3), 339–351.

Farabee, D., Wallisch, L., & Maxwell, J. C. (1995). Substance use among Texas Hispanics and non-Hispanics: Who's using, who's not, and why. *Hispanic Journal of Behavioral Sciences, 17*(4), 523–536.

Felix-Ortiz, M., Newcomb, M. D., & Myers, H. (1994). A multidimensional measure of cultural identity for Latino and Latina adolescents. *Hispanic Journal of Behavioral Sciences, 16*(2), 99–115.

Fernandez-Pol, B., Bluestone, H., Missouri, C., Morales, G., & Mizruchi, M. S. (1986). Drinking patterns of inner-city black Americans and Puerto Ricans. *Journal of Studies on Alcohol, 47*(2), 156–160.

Fernandez-Pol, B., Bluestone, H., Morales, G., & Mizruchi, M. (1985). Cultural influences and alcoholism: A study of Puerto Ricans. *Alcoholism: Clinical & Experimental Research, 9*(5), 443–446.

Fingarette, H. (1989). *Heavy drinking: The myth of alcoholism as a disease.* Berkeley: University of California Press.

Fitzpatrick, J. (1987). *Puerto Rican Americans: The meaning of migration to the mainland* (2nd ed.). Englewood Cliffs, NJ: Prentice Hall.

Frank, B., Schmeidler, J., Marel, R., & Maranda, M. (1988). *Illicit substance use among Hispanic adults in New York State.* New York: Division of Substance Abuse Services.

Ghali, S. B. (1982). Understanding Puerto Rican traditions. *Social Work, January,* 98-102.

Gil, R. M., & Vazquez, C. I. (1996). *The Maria paradox: How Latinas can merge old world traditions with new world self esteem.* New York: G. P. Putnam's Sons.

Gilbert, J. M. (1985). Alcohol-related practices, problems, and norms among Mexican Americans: An overview. *In Alcohol use among US ethnic minorities: Proceedings of a conference on the epidemiology of alcohol use and abuse among ethnic minority groups. Research Monograph No. 18* (pp. 115–134). Washington, DC: US Department of Health and Human Services.

Gilbert, J. M., & Cervantes, R. C. (1986). Patterns and practices of alcohol use among Mexican Americans: A comprehensive review. *Hispanic Journal of Behavioral Sciences, 8*(1), 1–60.

Glazer, N., & Moynihan, D. P. (1963). *Beyond the melting pot: The Negroes, Puerto Ricans, Jews, Italians, and Irish of New York City.* Cambridge, MA: MIT Press.

Gloria, A. M., & Peregoy, J. J. (1996). Counseling Latin alcohol and other substance users/abusers: Cultural considerations of counselors. *Journal of Substance Abuse Treatment, 13*(2), 119–126.

Goode, E. (1989). *Drugs in American society* (3rd ed.). New York: McGraw-Hill.

Graves, T. D. (1967). Acculturation, access, and alcohol in a tri-ethnic community. *American Anthropologist, 69,* 306–321.

Gurin, G. (1986). Drinking Behavior, Norms, and Problems in Puerto Rican Adults: A Proposal Submitted to Department of Health and Human Services. New York.

Harmon, M. P., Castro, F. G., & Coe, K. (1996). Acculturation and cervical cancer: Knowledge, beliefs, and behaviors of Hispanic women. *Women & Health, 24*(3), 37–58.

Heather, N., & Robinson, I. (1981). *Controlled drinking.* London: Methuen.

Hirschi, T. (1969). *Causes of delinquency.* Berkeley, CA: University of California Press.

Hoffman, F. (1994). Cultural adaptation of Alcoholics Anonymous to serve Hispanic populations. *International Journal of the Addictions, 29*(4), 445–460.

Jellinek, E. M. (1960). *The disease concept of alcoholism.* New Haven, CT: College and University Press.

Johnson, L. V., & Matre, M. (1978). Anomie and alcohol use drinking patterns in Mexican American and Anglo neighborhoods. *Journal of Studies on Alcohol, 39*(5), 894–902.

Kendall, P. L., & Wolf, K. M. (1957). The two purposes of deviant case analysis. In P. F. Lazarsfeld & M. Rosenberg (Eds.), *The language of social research* (pp. 167–170). Glencoe, IL: Free Press.

Kishline, A. (1994). *Moderate drinking: The moderation management guide for people who want to reduce their drinking.* New York: Three Rivers Press.

Klein, J. (1976). Ethnotherapy with Jews. *International Journal of Mental Health, 5*(2), 26–38.

Klein, J. W. (1980). *Jewish identity and self-esteem: Healing wounds through ethnotherapy.* New York: The American Jewish Committee.

Kranau, E. J., Green, V., & Valencia-Weber, G. (1982). Acculturation and the Hispanic woman: Attitudes toward women, sex-role attribution, sex-role behavior, and demographics. *Hispanic Journal of Behavioral Sciences, 4*(1), 21–40.

Krause, N., & Van Tran, T. (1989). Stress and religious involvement among older blacks. *Journal of Gerontology: Social Sciences, 44,* 4–13.

Lafferty, N. A., Holden, J. M., & Klein, H. E. (1980). Norm qualities and alcoholism. *International Journal of Social Psychiatry, 26,* 159–165.

LaFromboise, T., Coleman, H. L., & Gerton, J. (1993). Psychological impact of biculturalism: Evidence and theory. *Psychological Bulletin, 114*(3), 395–412.

Larsen, D. E., & Abu-Laban, B. (1968). Norm qualities and deviant drinking behavior. *Social Problems, 15*(4), 441–450.

Laureano, M., & Poliandro, E. (1991). Understanding cultural values of Latino male alcoholics and their families: A culture sensitive model. Special issue: Chemical dependency: Theoretical approaches and strategies working with individuals and families. *Journal of Chemical Dependency Treatment, 4*(1), 137–155.

Lewin, K. (1948). *Resolving social conflicts.* New York: Harper & Row.

Lewis, J. A., Dana, R. Q., & Blevins, G. A. (1988). *Substance abuse counseling: An individualized approach.* Belmont, CA: Brooks/Cole.

Lieberman, L. (1987). Jewish alcoholism and the disease concept. *Journal of Psychology and Judaism, 11*(3), 165–180.

Linsky, A. S., Colby, J. P., Jr., & Straus, M. A. (1986). Drinking norms and alcohol-related problems in the United States. *Journal of Studies on Alcohol, 47*(3), 384–393.

Lovato, C. Y., Litrownik, A. J., Elder, J., & Nunez-Liriano, A. (1994). Cigarette and alcohol use among migrant Hispanic adolescents. *Family & Community Health, 16*(4), 18–31.

Madsen, W. (1964). The alcoholic agringado. *American Anthropologist, 66,* 355–361.

Maldonado-Sierra, E. D., Trent, R. D., & Marina, R. F. (1960). Neurosis and traditional family beliefs in Puerto Rico. *International Journal of Social Psychiatry, VI*(3 & 4), 237–246.

Mann, L. (1987). *Ethnotherapy with Italian-Americans: An evaluation of short-term, group exploration of ethnic identification and self-esteem.* Unpublished doctoral dissertation, New York University, New York.

Maril, R. L., & Zavaleta, A. N. (1979). Drinking patterns of low-income Mexican American women. *Journal of Studies on Alcohol, 40*(5), 480–484.

Marin, G. (1996). Expectancies for drinking and excessive drinking among Mexican Americans and non-Hispanic whites. *Addictive Behaviors, 21*(4), 491–507.

Marin, G., & Posner, S. F. (1995). The role of gender and acculturation on determining the consumption of alcoholic beverages among Mexican-

Americans and Central Americans in the United States. *International Journal of the Addictions, 30*(7), 779–794.

Markides, K. S., Krause, N., & Mendes de Leon, C. F. (1988). Acculturation and alcohol consumption among Mexican Americans: A three generation study. *American Journal of Public Health, 78*(9), 1178–1181.

Merton, R. K. (1968). *Social theory and social structure.* New York: Free Press.

Mirage, L. W. (1987). *Valence of ethnicity, perception of discrimination, and self-esteem in high risk minority college students.* Unpublished doctoral dissertation, Fordham University, New York.

Montijo, J. (1975). The Puerto Rican client. *Professional Psychology: Research & Practice, 6*(4), 475–477.

Natera, G., Herrejon, M. E., & Casco, M. (1988). Locus of control in couples with different patterns of alcohol consumption. *Drug & Alcohol Dependence, 22*(3), 179–186.

Neff, J. A. (1993). Life stressors, drinking patterns, and depressive symptomatology: Ethnicity and stress-buffer effects of alcohol. *Addictive Behaviors, 18*(4), 373–387.

Neff, J. A., & Hoppe, S. K. (1993). Race, ethnicity, acculturation, and psychological distress: Fatalism and religiosity as cultural resources. *Journal of Community Psychology, 21*(1), 3–20.

Neff, J. A., Hoppe, S. K., & Parea, P. (1987). Acculturation and alcohol use: Drinking patterns and problems among Anglo and Mexican-American male drinkers. *Hispanic Journal of Behavioral Sciences, 9*(2), 151–181.

Nespor, K. (1985). Stressful life events: A preventive approach. *International Journal of Psychosomatics, 32*(4), 28–32.

Olmstead, R. E., Guy, S. M., O'Mally, P. M., & Bentler, P. M. (1991). Longitudinal assessment of the relationship between self-esteem, fatalism, loneliness, and substance use. *Journal of Social Behavior & Personality, 6*(4), 749–770.

Oquendo, M. A. (1994). Differential diagnosis of ataque de nervios. *American Journal of Orthopsychiatry, 63*(1), 60–65.

Padilla, A. M. (Ed.). (1980). *Acculturation: Theory, models and some new findings.* Boulder, CO: Westview Press for the Advancement of Science.

Padilla, E. (1958). *Up from Puerto Rico.* New York: Columbia University Press.

Page, J. B., Rio, L., Sweeney, J., & McKay, C. (1985). Alcohol and adaptation to exile in Miami's Cuban population. In L. Bennett & G. Ames (Eds.), *The*

American experience with alcohol: Contrasting cultural perspectives (pp. 315–332). New York: Plenum Press.

Panitz, D. R., McConchie, R. D., Sauber, S. R., & Fonseca, J. A. (1983). The role of machismo and the Hispanic family in the etiology and treatment of alcoholism in Hispanic American males. *American Journal of Family Therapy, 11*(1), 31–44.

Park, R. E., & Miller, H. A. (1921). *Old world traits transplanted.* New York: Harper Brothers.

Passalacqua, J. M. G. (1994). The Puerto Ricans: Migrants or commuters? In C. A. Torre, H. Rodriquez Vecchini, & W. Burgos (Eds.), *The commuter nation: Perspectives on Puerto Rican migration* (pp. 103–113). Rio Piedras, Puerto Rico: Editorial de la Universidad de Puerto Rico.

Peck, S. (1990). *Foreword. In H. Lewis, A question of values.* San Francisco: Harper & Row.

Peele, S. (1985). *The meaning of addiction: Compulsive experience and its interpretation.* Lexington, MA: Lexington Books.

Peele, S. (1989). *Diseasing of America: Addiction treatment out of control.* Lexington, MA: Lexington Books.

Perez, R., Padilla, A. M., Ramirez, A., Ramirez, R., & Rodriguez, M. (1980). Correlates and changes over time in drug and alcohol use within a barrio population. *American Journal of Community Psychology, 8*(6), 621–636.

Pittman, D. J. (1967). International overview: Social and cultural factors in drinking patterns, pathological and nonpathological. In D. J. Pittman (Ed.), *Alcoholism* (pp. 3–20). New York: Harper & Row.

Purdy, B. A., Simari, C. G., & Colon, G. (1983). Religiosity, ethnicity, and mental health: Interface the 80s. *Counseling & Values, 27*(2), 112–122.

Quayle, D., & Medved, D. (1996). *The American family: Discovering the values that make us strong.* New York: Harper Collins.

Quiles, J. A. (1989). The cultural assimilation and identity transformation of Hispanics: A conceptual paradigm. ERIC Microfiche Number: ED315473.

Quintero, G., & Estrada, A. L. (1998). "Machismo," drugs and street survival in a US–Mexico border community. *Free Inquiry in Creative Sociology, 26*(1), 3–10.

Rachal, J. V., Williams, J. R., Brehm, M. L., Cavanaugh, B., Moore, R. P., & Eckerman, W. C. (1975). *A national study of adolescent drinking behavior, attitudes and correlates* (PB-246-002). Washington, DC: National Institute on Alcohol Abuse and Alcoholism.

Ramirez, J. I., & Hosch, H. M. (1991). The influence of acculturation on family functioning among Hispanic Americans in a bicultural community. Tempe, AZ. ERIC Microfiche Number: ED346387.

Ramirez, R. R. (2000). *The Hispanic population in the United States: Population characteristics* (P20-527). Washington, DC: US Census Bureau.

Ready, T. (1991). Latino immigrant youth: Passages from adolescence to adulthood. ERIC Microfiche Number: ED363672.

Robinson, L. (1998). Hispanics' don't exist, *US News Online.* http://www.usnews.com/usnews/issue/980511/11hisp.htm.

Rodriguez, S. (1995). Hispanics in the United States: An insight into group characteristics. www.hhs.gov/about/heo/hgen.html: Department of Health and Human Services.

Rodriquez-Andrew, S. (1998). Alcohol use and abuse among Latinos: Issues and examples of culturally competent services. In M. Delgado (Ed.), *Alcohol use/abuse among Latinos: Issues and examples of culturally competent services* (pp. 55–66). New York: Haworth Press.

Rogler, L. H., & Santana Cooney, R. (1994). From Puerto Rico to New York City. In C. A. Torre, H. Rodriquez Vecchini, & W. Burgos (Eds.), *The commuter nation: Perspectives on Puerto Rican migration* (pp. 187–220). Rio Piedras, Puerto Rico: Editorial de la Universidad de Puerto Rico.

Rosado, J. W. (1980). Important psychocultural factors in the delivery of mental health services to lower-class Puerto Rican clients: A review of recent studies. *Journal of Community Psychology, 8*(3), 215–226.

Rosenberg, M. (1968). *The logic of survey analysis.* New York: Basic Books.

Ross, C. E., Mirowsky, J., & Cockerham, W. C. (1983). Social class, Mexican culture, and fatalism: Their effects on psychological distress. *American Journal of Community Psychology, 11*(4), 383–399.

Rosten, L. (1965). *The education of H*Y*M*A*N K*A*P*L*A*N.* New York: Harcourt Brace Jovanovich.

Rothenberg, A. (1964). Puerto Rico and aggression. *American Journal of Psychiatry, 120,* 962–970.

Rudy, D. R. (1986). *Becoming alcoholic: Alcoholics Anonymous and the reality of alcoholism.* Carbondale and Edwardsville: Southern Illinois University Press.

Ruef, A. M., Litz, B. T., & Schlenger, W. E. (2000). Hispanic ethnicity and risk for combat-related posttraumatic stress disorder. *Cultural Diversity & Ethnic Minority Psychology, 6*(3), 235–251.

Ruiz, A. S. (1984). Cross-cultural group counseling and the use of the sentence completion method. *Journal for Specialists in Group Work, 9*(3), 131–136.

Salvo, J. J., Ortiz, R. J., & Lobo, A. P. (1994). *Puerto Rican New Yorkers in 1990* (Report DCP 94-09). New York: Department of City Planning.

Sanchez-Dirks, R. D. (1978). *Hispanic drinking practices: A comparative study of Hispanic and Anglo adolescent drinking patterns.* Unpublished Dissertation, New York University, New York.

Sandoval, M. C., & De la Roza, M. C. (1986). A cultural perspective for serving the Hispanic client. In H. P. Lefley & P. B. Pedersen (Eds.), *Cross-cultural training for mental health professionals* (pp. 151–181). Springfield, IL: Charles C. Thomas.

Santiago-Irizarry, V. (1996). Culture as cure. *Cultural Anthropology, 11*(1), 2–24.

Santiago-Rivera, A. L. (1995). Developing a culturally sensitive treatment modality for bilingual Spanish speaking clients incorporating language and culture in counseling. *Journal of Counseling and Development, 74*(1), 12–17.

Schutz, A. (1944). The stranger: An essay in social psychology. *American Journal of Sociology, XLIX* (6), 499–507.

Sellin, T. (1938). Culture conflict and crime. *American Journal of Sociology, 44,* 97–103.

Shils, E. (1981). *Tradition.* Boston, MA: Faber and Faber.

Singer, M. (1984). Spiritual healing and family therapy: Common approaches to the treatment of alcoholism. *Family Therapy, 11*(2), 155–162.

Skolnick, J. H. (1958). Religious affiliation and drinking behavior. *Quarterly Journal of Studies on Alcoholism, 19,* 452–470.

Soto, E. (1983). Sex-role traditionalism and assertiveness in Puerto Rican women living in the United States. *Journal of Community Psychology, 11*(4), 346–354.

Spence, J. T., & Helmreich, R. L. (1972). The attitudes toward women scale: An objective instrument to measure attitudes toward the rights and roles of women in contemporary society. *Journal of Supplement Abstract Service, 2,* 66–72.

Stevens, E. P. (1973). Machismo and marianismo. *Society, 10*(86), 57–63.

Stonequist, E. V. (1937). *The marginal man: A study in personality and culture conflict*. New York: Charles Scribner's Sons.

Suarez, S. A., Fowers, B. J., Garwood, C. S., & Szapocznik, J. (1997). Biculturalism, differentness, loneliness, and alienation in Hispanic college students. *Hispanic Journal of Behavioral Sciences, 19*(4), 489–505.

Suchman, E. A. (1967). Preventive health behavior: A model for research on community health campaigns. *Journal of Health & Social Behavior, 8*(3), 197–209.

Szalay, L. B., Canino, G., & Vilov, S. K. (1993). Vulnerabilities and cultural change: Drug use among Puerto Rican adolescents in the United States. *International Journal of the Addictions, 28*(4), 327–354.

Terrell, M. D. (1993). Ethnocultural factors and substance abuse: Toward culturally sensitive treatment models. Special series: Psychosocial treatment of the addictions. *Psychology of Addictive Behaviors, 7*(3), 162–167.

Theodore, R. M. (1992). The relationship between locus of control and level of violence in married couples. In E. C. Vianno (Ed.), *Intimate violence: Interdisciplinary perspectives* (pp. 37–48). New York: Hemisphere.

Theodorson, G. A., & Theodorson, A. G. (1969). *A modern dictionary of sociology*. New York: Thomas Y. Crowell.

Tonigan, J. S., Connors, G. J., & Miller, W. R. (1998). Special populations in Alcoholics Anonymous. *Alcohol Health & Research World, 22*(4), 281–285.

Torre, C. A., Rodriquez Vecchini, H., & Burgos, W. (1994). *The commuter nation: Perspectives on Puerto Rican migration*. Rio Piedras, Puerto Rico: Editorial de la Universidad de Puerto Rico.

Trice, H. M., & Roman, P. M. (1970). Delabeling, relabeling and Alcoholics Anonymous. *Social Problems, 17*, 468–480.

Trice, H. M., & Roman, P. M. (1978). *Spirits and demons at work: Alcohol and other drugs on the job* (2nd ed.). Ithaca, NY: Cornell University.

Trimpey, J. (1989). *The small book: A revolutionary alternative for overcoming alcohol and drug dependence*. New York: Delacorte Press.

Trotter, R. T. (1985). Mexican-American experience with alcohol. South Texas examples. In L. Bennett & G. Ames (Eds.), *The American experience with alcohol: Contrasting cultural perspectives* (pp. 279–296.). New York: Plenum Press.

Ullman, A. D. (1958). Sociocultural backgrounds of alcoholism. *The Annals of the American Academy of Political and Social Sciences, 315*, 48–54.

United States Census Bureau. (1999). US Hispanic Population: 1999. www.census.gov/population/socdemo/hispanic/cps99/99show.ppt.

Valdez, J. N. (2000). Psychotherapy with bicultural Hispanic clients. *Psychotherapy, 37*(3), 240–246.

Vazquez-Nuttall, E., Avila-Vivas, Z., & Morales-Barreto, G. (1984). Working with Latin American families. In J. C. Hansen & B. F. Okun (Eds.), *Family therapy with school related problems: The family therapy collections* (Vol. 9, pp. 74–90). Rockville: Aspen.

Vazquez-Nuttall, E., Romero-Garcia, I., & DeLeon, B. (1987). Sex role and perceptions of femininity and masculinity of Hispanic women. *Psychology of Women Quarterly, 11*, 409–425.

Vega, W. A., Alderete, E., Kolody, B., & Aguilar-Gaxiola, S. (1998). Illicit drug use among Mexicans and Mexican Americans in California: The effects of gender and acculturation. *Addiction, 93*(12), 1839–1850.

Vega, W. A., Gil, A. G., Warheit, G. J., Zimmerman, R. S., & Apospori, E. (1993). Acculturation and delinquent behavior among Cuban American adolescents: Toward an empirical model. *American Journal of Community Psychology, 21*(1), 113-125.

Velez, C. N., & Ungemack, J., A. (1989). Drug use among Puerto Rican youth: An exploration of generational status differences. *Social Science Medicines, 29*(6), 779–789.

Velez-Blasini, C. J. (1997). A cross-cultural comparison of alcohol expectancies in Puerto Rico and the United States. *Psychology of Addictive Behaviors, 11*(2), 124–141.

Wagner-Echeagaray, F. A., Schutz, C. G., Chilcoat, H. D., & Anthony, J. C. (1994). Degree of acculturation and the risk of crack cocaine smoking among Hispanic Americans. *American Journal of Public Health, 84*(11), 1825-1827.

Wargacki, J. M. (1986). Assimilation and educational determinants for Puerto Rican children (Vol. 23). ERIC Microfiche Number: ED280747.

Weil, A. (1986). *The natural mind: An investigation of drugs and the higher consciousness* (rev. ed.). Boston: Houghton Mifflin.

Wheaton, R. B. (1983). Stress, personal coping resources, and psychiatric symptoms: An investigation of interactive models. *Journal of Health & Social Behavior, 24*(3), 208–229.

Wilsnack, R. W., & Wilsnack, S., C. (1978). Sex roles and drinking among adolescent girls. *Journal of Studies on Alcohol, 39*(11), 1855–1874.

Winthrop, R. H. (1991). *Dictionary of concepts in cultural anthropology.* New York: Greenwood Press.

Zangwill, I. (1913). *The melting-pot, drama in four acts.* New York: Macmillan.

INDEX

Abstinence
  attitudes, 137
  expectations, 123
  parents, 115–117
  rationales, 127–132
  women, 39, 88, 91, 150, 178–179
Abu-Laban, Baha, 148
Acculturation
  and attitudes, 142
  and gender, 54
  and traditionalism, 70, 73
  as explanation, 13–14, 43–44, 55,
    86, 88, 91–93, 95, 146–148,
    151–152, 156–158, 160, 157,
    170–173, 176, 179–183,
    186–186, 189
  measurement, 1, 23, 26–27,
    44–45, 47–50, 53–54, 148, 151
  modes of adaptation, 36–37, 41,
    90, 171, 183
  problems of, 12, 60–61

process of, 35–38, 40–42, 87, 91,
  150, 190
stress, 90, 94
Addiction, 21, 106, 110, 137, 140,
  143–144
Age, 19, 24, 27, 53–54, 74–75, 84,
  109–110, 115–116, 132, 136, 169,
  174–175
Aguilar-Gaxiola, Sergio, 43
Aguirre-Molina, Marilyn, 12, 42, 63,
  65, 85, 94, 99
Alcocer, Anthony, 42, 87, 146
Alcohol
  abuse, 92
  and abstainers, 160
  and Hispanics, 22–23, 25–26, 39,
    43, 85, 87
  attitudes, 115, 136
  etiology, 90
  expectancies, 122–125, 128–131
  function of, 83–84